The
New Culture
of
Therapeutic
Activity with
Older People

Titles in the **Speechmark Editions** series:

Accent Method: A Rational Voice Therapy in Theory & Practice, Kirsten Thyme-Frøkjær & Børge Frøkjær-Jensen

Beyond Aphasia: Therapies for Living with Communication Disability, Carole Pound, Susie Parr, Jayne Lindsay & Celia Woolf

Challenging Behaviour in Dementia: A person-centred approach, Graham Stokes

Counselling with Reality Therapy, Robert E Wubbolding & John Brickell

Elder Abuse: Therapeutic Perspectives in Practice, Andrew Papadopoulos & Jenny la Fontaine

Essential Dementia Care Handbook, edited by Graham Stokes & Fiona Goudie

Family Therapy with Older Adults & their Families, Alison Marriott

Head Injury: A Practical Guide, Trevor Powell

Human Communication: A Linguistic Introduction, Graham Williamson

Manual of AAC Assessment, Arlene McCurtin & Geraldine Murray

The New Culture of Therapeutic Activity with Older People, edited by Tessa Perrin

Person-Centred Approaches to Dementia Care, Ian Morton

Teamwork: A Guide to Successful Collaboration in Health & Social Care, Sue Hutchings, Judy Hall & Barbara Lovelady

The
New Culture
of
Therapeutic
Activity with
Older People

edited by
Tessa Perrin

Speechmark

Speechmark Publishing Ltd
Telford Road, Bicester, Oxon OX26 4LQ, UK

First published in 2004 by
Speechmark Publishing Ltd, Telford Road, Bicester, Oxon OX26 4LQ, United Kingdom
Tel: +44 (0)1869 244 644 Fax: +44 (0)1869 320 040
www.speechmark.net

002-5142/Printed in the United Kingdom/3000

British Library Cataloguing in Publication Data
Perrin, Tessa
   The new culture of therapeutic activity with older people. – (Speechmark Editions)
   1. Occupational therapy for the aged   2. Aged – Care – Philosophy
   I. Perrin, Tessa
   615.8'515'0846

ISBN-10: 0 86388 442 3
ISBN-13: 978 0 86388 442 9

Contents

List of contributors   vii

Foreword by Graham Stokes   xi

Introduction   xv

1 Towards a New Culture   1
Tessa Perrin

2 The Developing Culture in its Political Context   18
Rosemary Hurtley

3 The Unit Manager: The Key to Cultural Change   38
Keena Millar and Sylvie Silver

4 The Unit Manager: Creating a Positive Influence   54
Paul Smith

5 Successful Activity Planning   71
Hazel May

6 The Critical Importance of Biographical Knowledge   88
Charlie Murphy

7 The Activity Coordinator: On the Way In or
On the Way Out?   104
Vivienne Ratcliffe

8 Providing Activities in Residential Care Settings:
Dilemmas for Staff   119
Kenneth Hawes

9 Activity Training in the New Culture   135
Tessa Perrin

10 Activity Provision and Community Care:
The Harlow Experience   147
Helen Crumpton

11 Activity Provision and Community Care:
The Leicester Experience   167
*Caroline Ryder-Jones, Wendy Ferguson and
Rebecca Colledge*

12 Changing a Culture: The Westminster Project   186
Richard Mepham

13 Collaborative Networking and Community
Development: The Way Forward   204
Sally Knocker

14 NAPA: Steering the Path from Entertainer to
Reflective Practitioner   218
Simon Labbett

References   229

Index   234

Contributors

Rebecca Colledge is a Senior 1 occupational therapist for Leicestershire Partnership NHS Trust. After qualifying in 1992 Rebecca worked in physical medicine. Since 1994 she has worked in a community mental health team in mental health services for older people.

Helen Crumpton achieved a BA (Hons) in Interdisciplinary Human Studies from Bradford University, and has undertaken extensive dementia care training. She is the manager of Merefield Day Centre in Harlow, a specialist day-care facility for older people with mental health needs. During her seven years at Merefield Helen has established an innovative outreach service taking specialist day-care activities into people's own homes. She is also an active volunteer for the local Alzheimer's Society.

Wendy Ferguson is a Senior 1 occupational therapist for Leicestershire Partnership NHS Trust and is currently working in a community mental health team for older people.

Kenneth Hawes works as an Assistant Care Manager with older people for Westminster Social and Community Services. He has spent many years working as an Activities Officer in residential care where he was involved in a number of innovative projects for older people. He also takes a special interest in management issues and staff welfare.

Rosemary Hurtley, Dip COT, SROT, MA, has worked as an occupational therapist in the NHS, private, voluntary and statutory services. She specialises in the care of older people and quality of life, and also as a consultant in long-term care. Rosemary is a trustee of NAPA and has taught on the NAPA course leading to the City & Guilds Certificate in Providing Therapeutic Activities for Older People. She is also co-author of *The Successful Activity Co-ordinator*.

Sally Knocker, Pg Dp Dramatherapy, works part time for NAPA as the Growing with Age national project manager, and part time as a trainer in dementia care and promoting activity with older people. She recently wrote and edited the *Alzheimer's Society Book of Activities*. Sally has worked for 15 years in the dementia care field as a development worker with the Alzheimer's Society, and as a dementia specialist trainer in a social services department before training as a dramatherapist.

Simon Labbett is community arts officer with the Royal National Institute of the Blind (RNIB). He is currently Chairman of NAPA and, in what time remains, he is a musician.

Hazel May is a state registered occupational therapist with a master's degree in philosophy and healthcare. She works independently as a dementia care therapist, consultant and trainer from her home base in Wiltshire. Currently she works in association with the Bradford Dementia Group and Dementia Voice in Bristol, in addition to developing dementia care services at the Royal Hospital Chelsea, the Milestones Trust in Bristol and the Dorset NHS Trust.

Richard Mepham has a background in psychology and development in services for older adults. He has experience of promoting activity in both voluntary and statutory settings. He lives with his partner in South Wales and is employed by NAPA promoting access to training and education.

Keena Millar completed her registered general nurse training in Edinburgh in 1973. She also undertook an English Nursing Board course in elderly care in 1993, has a Diploma in Higher Education in Nursing Studies (2000) and a Diploma in Performance Coaching (2001). She was appointed deputy matron to a nursing home in 1988 and became matron later that year.

Charlie Murphy has worked as fieldworker for the voluntary sector at the Dementia Services Development Centre in Stirling since 1992. He regularly delivers training in life story work to groups of staff or family carers. His other interests include evaluating services for individuals with dementia and promoting the incorporation of service user views in service evaluations.

Tessa Perrin is a state registered occupational therapist with many years experience of working in residential and day-care settings for older people. She has a particular interest in the training of care staff and is Honorary Director of Training for NAPA. She is author of numerous publications on activity-related matters.

Vivienne Ratcliffe has had over 20 years diverse experience of both caring and support for carers. Eight years in a nursing home for dementia provided the core experience related in her chapter, supplemented by continuing voluntary work for the elderly and others with disabilities and dementia-related illnesses.

Caroline Ryder-Jones worked in Leicester from 1992 to 2001, specialising in community mental health for people over 65 years of age. She currently works in a young onset dementia team within the Tees and North East Yorkshire Trust.

Sylvie Silver has worked as a nursing auxiliary, ward clerk and special needs classroom assistant. She has also managed a day service for adults with learning difficulties and has spent the last seven years as Leisure Services Manager providing activities in a nursing home for older people. She has a Diploma in Performance Coaching (2003), and recently achieved the City & Guilds 6977 Certificate in Providing Therapeutic Activities for Older People.

Paul Smith qualified in 1983 as an RMN. He has since studied psychotherapy, group psychotherapy and clinical hypnotherapy. He has worked as charge nurse within the NHS, as home manager, senior home manager and troubleshooter in the independent sector. He is now regional manager for European Care Ltd (UK).

Foreword

IN THE UNITED KINGDOM the number of people over 85 years old is projected to rise by 79 per cent between 1995 and 2031, and one consequence of our ageing society will be an increasing requirement to meet the needs of the minority of older adults with chronic illness and disability. More and more people with dependency needs are living, and will continue to live, in either their own homes with family and/or domiciliary support, or will be accommodated in supported independent living arrangements. This social care initiative will, in the short term, offset the loss of 60,000 beds in the long-stay care sector that has occurred over the past five years. There will, however, also be an increasing demand for care home provision in order to meet the requirements of older people whose needs are complex and challenging. Needs that are characterised by severity, risk and unpredictability. One conservative estimate is that the number of older people in long-term care will rise to 670,000 by 2031, of whom those with cognitive impairment will number 365,000.

Care homes are providing modernised long-stay healthcare that is concerned with the management of chronic disease. When an older person enters a care home, added value is traditionally measured in terms of palliative healthcare gain, a safe care setting and functional improvement. This cannot, however, be the limit of our vision for long-term care. Admission to a care home should be seen as a positive step on the spectrum of dependency – ideally core care needs will not only be met, but there will also be equal regard for the person and the quality of life to be lived. There will be reasons to get up in the morning, one day will differ from another, and there will be much to look forward to – all this imbued with a sense that the individual matters. Yet, time and time again, the poor quality of life for older people in care settings has been documented. Loneliness and the loss of activity and purpose have been identified as aspects of institutional life. The characteristic activity of older people in care settings is inactivity! Doing nothing or sleeping prevail. If it is unthinkable for us to spend hour after hour staring at the wall opposite, exposed to little other than a fluorescent light and bemusing background noise, how can such a malign process be appropriate to the needs of older people in care settings? Terms such as 'institutional maintenance' and 'conveyor belt care' have been used to describe the procedures and routines that benefit the smooth running of the institution, rather than the needs of those who live in them. The outcome is that we observe people living lives without meaning.

Many contemporary providers of care aspire to deliver environments that meet, rather than frustrate, the needs of their clients and residents. Hence this volume is a timely and valuable contribution, both to the promotion of therapeutic activity with older people, and the need to articulate the role and value of activity practitioners. The book's principle message is that the provision of activity in care settings is a healthcare essential, and hence that there is a moral obligation to deliver activity lifestyles. Activity is not the icing on the cake, it is a fundamental recipe ingredient.

The book's editor, Tessa Perrin, has herself contributed two chapters, and brings to the work a wealth of experience in occupational therapy and activity provision, both as practitioner and educator. She has developed special interests in the genesis of behaviour and the delivery of need-appropriate activity in dementia care, and her expertise and vision are effectively distilled in the structure and content of this book. It is pleasing to read so much on how people with dementia can be supported in the pursuit of purposeful and enjoyable experiences. Traditionally the inverse care law has reigned supreme – those who are most cognitively disabled receive least support from practitioners; while those who are most cognitively able, and who thus have the capacity to be self-motivating, receive the most encouragement and guidance!

The New Culture of Therapeutic Activity with Older People sees the coming together of a number of committed and visionary professionals from a variety of backgrounds who are convinced of the therapeutic value of activities with older people. They endeavour to define the benchmarks of what an activity culture is, and what an activity therapist and provider does; moreover they wish to evolve and support the 'fledgling profession' of activity specialist, in the words of one contributor. It is acknowledged that activity professionals need to be trained, and their skills and knowledge valued by colleagues, so that they are not seen as peripheral members of the care team, but are instead regarded as key practitioners in healthcare delivery.

This book offers a unique contribution in that, as well as identifying the challenges facing activity workers, it also provides a theoretical foundation for what is meant by therapeutic activity. It is not an activity manual, but a body of work that places activity in the context of principles and good practice, resonating with the need to be person-centred in all that is planned and provided. Chapters that are clearly and entertainingly written draw on real and personal experience to elucidate the influence of contextual factors: in particular the role of the home or unit manager, who most often sets the cultural tone, can act as an agent of change, and provides, through example, leadership. The service projects described are deeply revealing, and succeed in communicating the challenges faced by anyone who wishes to drive forward activity cultures that truly impact on people's lives.

In the new culture of therapeutic activity, purposeful engagement has inspiring goals: engendering feelings of fulfilment, happiness and achievement; encouraging activities that only happen in groups and at certain times of day; and valuing individual work that can be planned, spontaneous, or embedded in the activities of daily living. Nor is direct practice the preserve of any single profession or discipline. All who have contact with older people in receipt of care have the potential to take responsibility for the enrichment of a person's life. Yet, for this to happen, it is argued that managers must action a culture that neither explicitly nor implicitly conveys the message that care standards are governed by task performance; a culture that respects the workloads carried by care staff, and appreciates that if the needs of carers are not met, the motivation to meet in full the needs of their residents or clients may be absent.

Each chapter contributes to the weaving of a tapestry that successfully integrates vision, theory and practice. Managers and practitioners alike who wish to invest in the meaningful provision of activities will benefit from their own investment of time in reading this book. Its scope makes it relevant to all care settings aspiring to add value to people's lives by giving opportunity for therapeutic activity.

The subject of this book is of increasing public importance. We no longer measure the value of care solely by how well physical needs are met, and how decline is managed. Instead, commissioners, providers and inspectors are motivated to seek the provision of fulfilling lifestyles that truly reveal a life that is worth living. I warmly recommend this book to all people engaged in the delivery of quality care settings for older people.

Graham Stokes
Consultant Clinical Psychologist
Head of Mental Health, BUPA Care Homes

Introduction

THE LAST TEN YEARS have seen a dramatic and very welcome increase in the range of activity manuals on the market: books full of ideas about things to do with older people who live in care settings. In fact carers today now have a veritable library to choose from in the matter of activity planning; a far healthier resource than was available when I first started working in this field close on twenty years ago, and one which reflects the care profession's growing concern with the quality of life of the older person in care.

Unfortunately, this picture also reflects the industry's preoccupation with 'ideas'. Most activity providers who come on training courses are pre-eminently concerned with ideas. They are not usually looking for principles, or theory, and many are not even concerned with good practice. They want 'new ideas', 'new things to do', 'quick and easy activities which don't require much preparation'. This is quite understandable, but a little disturbing. It is understandable because many, if not most, activity providers are under considerable pressure from team colleagues to produce visible evidence of as many clients as possible being involved in activity. Time constraints and inadequate staffing dictate that most activity provision be carried out with groups of clients, and an endemic lack of understanding of the activity organiser role determines that activity organisers are generally required to 'do it all'.

However, the picture is also disturbing because it indicates an entrenchment in values and attitudes which are both elderly and out of date themselves. It reflects a culture of activity provision (indeed a culture of care generally) which has failed to move on from the hierarchical and task-driven institutional regimes of earlier years. It also perpetuates an erroneous notion of what activity provision is all about.

In principle of course, there is nothing wrong with good ideas and quick tips for activities – in their place. But if this is the driving force of activity provision in the work place, it is missing the mark; and it is my observation that this is indeed the driving force of many activity programmes. It evokes a futile desperation among activity organisers to maintain the 'right' kind of profile within their care team, and in the wider scheme of things it promotes misunderstanding, it retards progress, it serves to impoverish the activity programme, and thus has a negative impact on the quality of life of the clients it purports to serve.

The reason for this 'missing the mark' is, I believe, the preponderance of good ideas over good theory in the media, the ready availability of glossy, easy-to-read activity manuals and the relative inaccessibility of quality information on the critical matter of occupation and health, either in the literature or in educational and training resources.

This book attempts in some measure to make good the deficit. It is not an activity manual; the activity provider will not find here a bright idea for something to do with the group tomorrow afternoon. Nor, strictly speaking, is it a guide to good practice; such a guide is available from Speechmark (forthcoming). This book does, without doubt, make a statement of good practice, but that is not its first purpose. Its prime concern is to clarify and illuminate the changes that have been taking place in the field of activity provision over recent years, to identify the forces which have shaped activity provision past and present, to highlight aspects of the journey which have contributed to our current clarity of vision and purpose and, not least, to offer a challenge to future practitioners.

It is our hope that this book will in some measure fill the gap and complement existing publications on the matter of activities and older people. Chapter 1 highlights the contrast between old and new cultures, not in the sense of 'this is how it was then, this is how it is now', but in a representation of old and new thinking, and the impact which that has upon practice. Chapter 2 sets the 'historical' scene, a necessary read for the enquirer concerned with the socio-political forces which have shaped (and are shaping) current national requirements for activity provision.

Chapters 3 and 4 are, in my view, the most important chapters in the book. The power and influence of the care setting manager cannot be underestimated. For better or worse, like it or not, the success or failure of activity provision in a care setting is the ultimate responsibility of the unit manager. These chapters illustrate why that is so.

Chapters 5 and 6 describe the critical preliminaries for successful activity planning. Odd as it may seem today, assessment has not traditionally been a feature of activity provision. Today however, in our move away from entertainment and towards therapy, it is an essential requirement, and it is unthinkable that we should plan interventions without it.

Chapters 7 and 8 consider the response of staff to the developing culture of activity provision. Chapter 7 examines the role of the activity provider, asking the very pertinent question whether the activity coordinator role is needful in the new culture, or whether the task of activity provision is best served by being shared across disciplines. Chapter 8 examines a rarely sought view of this question – that of the care assistant.

Chapter 9 discusses the nature of activity training in the new culture, suggesting that traditional methods are inadequate, and proposing a new model for a new culture.

Chapters 10 to 12 are accounts of recent projects which have been designed to promote the new culture of activity provision in different settings. Chapter 10 recounts the experiences of a Harlow day-care team which successfully extended its service of support and activity provision into clients' own homes. The Leicester experience described in Chapter 11 had similarities to the Harlow project in the matter of service delivery and positive outcomes, but its own uniquely interesting genesis. This was a project devised and led by occupational therapists. It offers an insight into the OT profession's continuing identity crisis and the difficulties of response to the whole area of chronic disability. These two chapters describe a long-awaited and much needed development in services to those older people who have dementia.

Chapter 12 describes the Westminster project, and is a heart-searching discussion of the very practical difficulties inherent in introducing new culture approaches into the residential sector.

Set in the context of the Growing With Age project, Chapter 13 discusses the critical importance of networking and collaborative endeavour, not just in enhancing activity provision on the shop floor, but also in promoting the public face of the new culture.

Chapter 14 concerns the work of the National Association for Providers of Activities for Older People (NAPA). NAPA is a charitable organisation whose sole business is to support the work of the activity provider. This chapter describes its mission and issues a challenge to all those who desire to promote activity provision in the UK.

There is a new profession developing in this country. As I write, I have just had to stop for a minute and consult my dictionary to ensure that I am using the right word. I am. It defines the term profession as 'a vocation, a calling, especially one requiring advanced knowledge or training in some branch of learning or science'. In my view, this definition very accurately describes the new culture of activity provision as it is developing in the UK. The new culture of activity provision is being defined and will be driven by those who have a consuming passion for what they do; by those with an absolute commitment to ensuring that the quality of life needs of the older people in their care are met. Without question, this is a profession which requires advanced knowledge and training; this is a healthcare specialism in its own right. It may not have been perceived as such in the past, but it certainly is now.

The new profession is in its infancy as yet. It is emerging from the very solid principles and traditions of occupational healthcare that existed in the early days of occupational therapy. It is being shaped and driven by shop-floor practitioners of all disciplines who understand the critical link between occupation and health, and who have an urgent concern to see activity provision adopted as a healthcare essential in its own right. We have a long way to go yet, but a positive and substantial start has been made. In shedding light on cultural changes, past and present, it is our hope that this book will also illuminate the way ahead.

Finally, I would like to thank all those who have contributed to the book, for their commitment and enthusiasm and for their willingness to be a small part of a larger whole. To underline the message of the last two chapters of the book, that is the way ahead. The way ahead is about networking, about sharing, about working together, about contributing our own individual skills and knowledge to the common endeavour. Please join with us.

Tessa Perrin

CHAPTER 1

Towards a New Culture

Tessa Perrin

IN 1995 A BOOK WAS PUBLISHED called *The New Culture of Dementia Care* (Kitwood and Benson). Its keynote chapter was written by Tom Kitwood, a psychology lecturer who has been credited with having instigated the first real challenge to the long dominant medical model of dementia and dementia care. Kitwood had a particular gift for taking that which most of us in health and social care have understood intuitively for many years, and giving it back to us in print with a vocabulary and language which crystallise and categorise issues of particular importance, thereby enabling us to raise them for open debate at all levels of the healthcare hierarchy. His chapter on the new culture of dementia care did just that, drawing an articulate contrast between different aspects of the changing culture of healthcare and dementia care: this is how it was then – this is how it is now.

For those of us who have been living through many of the changes in the changing culture, such clarity of illustration was enormously helpful, explaining many of the tensions that have existed in practice settings, facilitating dialogue and pointing a way towards excellence. It impressed me and helped me as a practising clinician and researcher, and my mind has returned to it frequently as I have started to marshal my thoughts on the new culture of activity provision. The culture surrounding the provision of activities in care settings has of course been subject to many of those influences which have altered the dynamics of dementia care. Of particular note is the relatively recent move towards a person-centred approach and individualised models of care. But, as a therapeutic approach in its own right, activity provision has a history of cultural change which is unique and which merits close attention from any healthcare professional whose remit touches upon it. Indeed, in these days of increased accountability (see Department of Health, National Minimum Standards, 2001, and National Service Framework, 2001), it is imperative that elder care practitioners have a clear understanding of what has taken place, and how it affects current developments and future requirements.

I make no apologies therefore for borrowing Kitwood's format for this chapter as I attempt to set out in as clear and concise a manner as possible the changes that have taken, or are taking, place in the transition from old to new.

1 Old Culture
Activities are important in the care of older people
I was tempted to write here 'activities are unimportant in the care of older people' as this is the prevailing message obtained over many decades of walking into care settings characterised by what my colleague, Rosemary Hurtley (Chapter 2), has described so graphically as the 'geriatric pageant in death row' – the lethargy, lassitude, depression and challenging behaviours with which we are all too familiar. Certainly there are some who have held this view; there are some who still hold this view, but I believe them to be in the minority. Much more common is the view that activities are important. There have been and are, I believe, few healthcare workers who would not today ascribe to the view that

activities are 'a good thing', the rationale commonly given being that 'it is important for people to keep busy'.

New Culture
Activities are essential in the care of older people

There is a world of difference between 'important' and 'essential'. That difference is demonstrated by the individual practitioner's commitment to ensuring activity provision in their care setting. The person who believes that activities are important will feel under some constraint to ensure that they are provided in the care setting. The person who understands that activities are essential will recognise a moral obligation to do so. The new culture of therapeutic activity is built around this key premise – that activity is essential to human health and well-being, and that to neglect activity provision leads to ill health and disability. There is a large bank of empirical research evidence now available to support this premise (Perrin 1997).

2 Old Culture
Activity provision is an expensive option in care settings for older people

This is a commonly held view that goes back decades and manifests itself in statements such as:

- we don't have enough staff
- staff don't have enough time
- we haven't got an activity coordinator
- we don't have a budget for activities

It is a view that usually stems from a failure to understand exactly what constitutes 'an activity', and is commonly held by the person whose idea of activity is the bingo session, the reminiscence group or the outing.

New Culture

Activities are not necessarily expensive and certainly not an option: they are an integral part of the care process

The new culture proposes that any care process which does not have activity provision as an integral feature is deficient. Indeed, it may even be understood as potentially abusive in witholding an essential therapy. My personal view is that the care setting which witholds therapeutic activity is as negligent as the care setting which witholds essential drugs. The effects take much longer to manifest themselves, but they are just as devastating.

The new culture also understands that providing activities is not necessarily a costly business. What cost is there to folding the laundry, having a hand massage, bringing in the milk, dead-heading the roses, listening to Perry Como, making a pot of tea, handing round the biscuits, feeding the budgie? These are activities, the stuff of our everyday living, and they are virtually cost free. Without question money helps and gives us a greater range of opportunities to offer, but the fact that we don't have a budget for activities should not stop us from making the most of the innumerable daily living activities that abound in the care setting.

3 Old Culture

The group activity programme is the key indicator of an effective activity culture

There is no question but that the average visitor to a care setting today is on the lookout for overt evidence of a group activity programme. This could be a whiteboard divided into days of the week, indicating that the hairdresser comes on Tuesday morning, bingo is on Wednesday afternoon and a tea dance is held on Friday. Or it could be the entertainment taking place in the living room, or the minibus just departing for a trip to the coast. Observing action taking place among groups of clients is usually enough to satisfy the undiscerning enquirer that a positive activity culture exists. It may, but it may not. Groups of clients doing things does not constitute evidence of good practice.

New Culture
Person-centred activity programmes for the individual are the key indicator of an effective activity culture

What the interested enquirer (such as the family of a prospective client) should be looking for in a care setting is evidence that a personalised activity programme for each client is being implemented. This means that somewhere in Mrs Jones' care plan is documented:

- a programme of those activities that she wishes or needs to engage in over the course of a day or week
- evidence of any therapeutic goals pursued
- dated records of the evaluation and monitoring of her engagement in those activities

This is not to say that the enquirer should expect to see a programme in which Mrs Jones is fully occupied for a 16-hour waking day. The extent of her engagement will depend upon Mrs Jones herself and the constraints of the care setting. But there should be evidence of weekly, and in some cases daily, monitoring and recording. This is the best evidence of best practice.

4 Old Culture
Activity is about providing entertainment

There is nothing wrong with entertainment; this is the starting point of activity provision in many care settings. It helps, and may well be therapeutic for some individuals under some circumstances, but if our activity culture is built upon entertainment only, it is gravely deficient.

New Culture

Activity is about therapy – that is, it is about offering challenges and engendering positive change in the individual

Activity is essential for physical and psychological health and well-being. People whose health and well-being are compromised through inactivity (for whatever reason) can recoup losses and reversals through re-engagement in meaningful and satisfying activity. Activity provision in care settings is about enabling people (as far as they so wish) to function better and to feel better. As a corollary, it is also about enabling people already in good health to maintain that health at an optimum level.

5 Old Culture

Activities are the remit of the occupational therapist or the specially trained activities organiser

It is true that traditionally the occupational therapist has taken the key responsibility for the matter of activity provision, in healthcare settings at any rate. This is not the case with residential or day-care settings where they have always been in comparatively short supply. They are a particularly rare commodity in residential and nursing homes.

With the drift of the occupational therapy profession away from chronic disability settings has come the emergence of a 'new' practitioner, the activities organiser, to make good the deficit. Few, however, are specially trained, for, to date, there has been little or no training available for those holding such a role. The United States and Australia have a higher education system leading to an award of 'diversional' or 'recreational' therapy, but in the UK there is, thus far, nothing similar. By far the greatest number of those holding an activities organiser role in Britain are unqualified and untrained.

New Culture
Activities should be within the remit of all disciplines in the care setting

The new culture contends that it does not require a specially trained person to engage people in activities. It *does* require a specially trained person to deliver effective therapeutic activity programmes, but any careworker with good interpersonal skills should be able to engage a client in an activity. If she cannot, then she should not be holding a care role, for engaging someone therapeutically in an activity is about people skills, not activity skills. It does not matter how the table is laid or the picture painted; it does matter that satisfaction and improved self-esteem in the client are the result.

There is no question but that, as things stand in the care world at present, most care settings do need a specially designated and trained person to lead and direct activity provision, and to ensure therapeutic efficacy. But it is a nonsense to expect such a person to take responsibility for all the person-to-person engaging of clients in activity. This must be shared across the team to be effective. It can indeed be very effective, embracing and utilising the broad range of skills and personal qualities that is the gift of any sizeable care team.

6 Old Culture
Activities organisers need a range of skills in arts and/or crafts

This is a common misconception of the old culture, and stems primarily from the view outlined in item five above: that the activities organiser is the person who does it all, therefore they need to be multiskilled to bring a wide range of activities to the task. This view has also led to the employment of specialists, such as professional artists and craftspeople. There is, of course, nothing intrinsically wrong with this, except where there has been an underpinning assumption that because a person is a professional artist (or whatever) they will automatically be a good activity provider. They may, but they may not; if they are not, then they could do more harm than good.

New Culture
First and foremost, activities organisers need a range of effective interpersonal skills

The activities organiser needs first to be a 'people person'; art and craft skills are very secondary. In fact, not having art and craft skills can often be a plus. Some of the best sessions I have participated in have been where the activity provider has come alongside the clients as a novice, having a basic grasp of an art or craft technique, but able to make and share mistakes and enjoy a laugh together. This creates a situation of low demand for the client who feels no requirement then to perform to any particular standard.

The activities organiser needs to know how to use activity therapeutically; that is, how to balance the demands of an activity with the skills and preferences of a client. So, while there is a need for the activities organiser to be able to recognise the demands of activities and their separate component parts, there is also a need to know the client sufficiently well to be able to match activity to client at any given time, and on each occasion to establish an environment in which that activity will be received. It is my personal view that this demands the highest level of interpersonal skills.

7 Old Culture
Activities are selected and planned by the activities organiser

The activities organiser is the 'specialist' and decides what activities are going to take place and when.

New Culture
Activities are selected, if not planned, by the client(s)

You and I do not, by and large, have our daily activities planned for us. We decide what we want to do, how, when and with whom – and we go and do it. This is the norm. In our care settings, we need to be working towards the norm, but it is undeniably the case that many people who have begun to disengage from activity through illness, trauma or disability almost always require some degree of assistance to re-engage. That assistance should never take the form of prescription (this is what I think you should do) by any care worker, no matter their discipline. It should always be a matter of negotiation with the client. (What would you like to do or achieve? What changes would you like to make? How can I best assist you?) Our interventions should always be client-led as far as possible.

Having said that, there are particular difficulties in achieving client-led interventions with people who have cognitive or mental health difficulties, and who may well be unable to indicate effectively choice and preference. It may be difficult with this client group, but it is certainly not impossible. It does require more of a trial and error approach, and depends much more on direct observation as a means of determining the satisfactory engagement and well-being of the client. But there is no question that even those who cannot use verbal means to articulate their feelings and wishes will invariably find non-verbal ways to do so.

8 Old Culture
The best/usual times for activities are 10.30 to 12.00 and 14.00 to 16.00
This is certainly true of an activity culture which operates mainly around group activities led by a designated activity provider. These are the times when most care settings are free from the distraction of meals, drug rounds, etc.

New Culture
The best/usual time for activities is at intervals across the 24-hour period
It is a fundamental premise of the new culture that any positive engagement with another or with the environment is an activity, and that

all members of a care team have a responsibility to assist clients in this matter. If this premise is at the heart of a care setting's culture, it will follow automatically that activities can take place at any time – bathtime, teatime, bedtime, etc. The care assistant who is engaging a client in a leisurely, sensory bath before bed is just as legitimately engaging that client in an activity as the activities organiser who involved her in a group quiz over morning coffee. To 'confine' activities to a couple of hours mid-morning and mid-afternoon is to place unhelpful constraints upon a culture, and delivers an erroneous message about what activity means. The Westminster Project (Chapter 12) threw up an amusing but rather sad illustration of this. Care staff were regularly observed rushing residents (and themselves) through the aftermath of lunch, washing-up and clearing away (all legitimate activities for residents to be involved in), in order to prepare for the formal 'activity hour', timetabled to happen every day between 2 and 3pm. The observer felt that a cloud descended every day at 2pm. Staff who were relaxed and comfortable while involving residents in everyday domestic tasks, wilted visibly under the imposed requirement to 'do activities', such as table games, quizzes and crafts.

A word needs to be added here about activities for people with dementia. An individual's clock goes fairly early in dementia. In earlier dementia it is worth investing time and energy in trying to retain a daily routine for a person. However, by the time a person is requiring residential care, chronological time has become largely irrelevant and the care setting needs to acknowledge this. Does it matter when Mr Jones sleeps? Surely it matters only if he is hurting himself or others with his unconventional sleep pattern. If he is not, activities at 1 or 2am are entirely appropriate – and, as a bonus, relieve staff during the busier daytime hours when Mr Jones is sleeping.

9 Old Culture
Any activity is better than no activity
Or, doing something is better than doing nothing. This is a myth that became prevalent in care settings around the 1970s and 1980s, as the clientele of the average care home became frailer and more dependent – and more disengaged. It represents an uneducated view that 'being busy' somehow confers healthful benefits, although little was understood at the time of the connection between occupation and health.

New Culture
Some activities can be counter-therapeutic and damaging to the individual
No activity is inherently good or bad, therapeutic or counter-therapeutic. 'Therapy' exists in a person's use of an activity to positive effect. An activity which is therapeutic for one individual may be quite the opposite for another. Whether it is therapeutic or not for a particular individual will depend upon a number of factors:

- the nature of the activity;
- the inherent demands of the activity;
- the retained abilities of the individual;
- the likes, personal preferences and motivation of the individual.

The skill of the therapist lies in a careful balancing of these factors (as far as possible in negotiation with the client) to ensure positive effect. An activity which is overly demanding of the retained abilities of the client, and/or which has little meaning, value or purpose for the client, is likely to be unproductive, and has a potential to be damaging and destructive.

10 Old Culture
Severely impaired people cannot do activities

This is a commonly held attitude which derives from a failure to understand exactly what constitutes an activity. Carers who make statements of this nature about their clients generally mean that they cannot engage in the game of dominoes, the craft or the reminiscence, or benefit from the outing.

New Culture
There is only a very small percentage of people in care settings who cannot engage in activities; these are those people who have been described as being in a vegetative condition

Severe impairment is no bar to engaging in activities. It is true that the range of opportunities for activity decreases with increasing impairment. It is also true that engaging the severely impaired person in activity requires an understanding of chronic disability and a greater creativity and commitment. But, given that greater application, there is no reason why the severely impaired person should not be satisfactorily engaged in an activity of their choosing such as listening to music, stirring a cake mix, having a massage, or shredding the office waste paper.

11 Old Culture
Activity provision must fund itself

Sadly, this has been a fact of life in many care settings over the years. Activity provision has been perceived as of so little value that no specific budget is designated. The underpinning attitude to this lack of resourcing is: 'If you want to do activities that's fine, but you will have to ensure that it generates its own funding'. This in turn has led to an activity culture which is built around the need to make its own money to survive (and is therefore reliant upon making 'products' to sell, such as crafts, preserves and baking). It has also placed considerable stress on willing staff who have more than enough to contend with in meeting clients' needs, without having the additional responsibility of fund-raising.

New Culture
Activity provision must be funded

Activity provision should never expect activity providers to fund their own work. Not only is it making an unreasonable demand on staff to take on this additional (and often arduous) role as fund-raiser, but it also exerts an insidious pressure on staff to channel their efforts in ways which may be inappropriate. So, if a unit can only survive by raising its own funds, there is a significant need to emphasise activities which result in saleable products. This considerably limits the range of occupational opportunities available. It also favours the able person who retains the ability to engage with end-product tasks, and has a potential to marginalise the less able person who can no longer engage constructively with objects and requires alternative interventions. In fact it subtly militates against the whole concept of person-centred therapeutic activity.

Having said that, there are some care settings where more able people can derive a very real sense of purpose and contribution from a conscious commitment to raising funds in such a way, and this can be enormously therapeutic in itself. But it doesn't alter the fact that forcing activity providers to fund themselves is wrong, and projects based on this principle will generally burn out in due course. Activity provision should be valued for the very significant healthcare contribution it makes and funded accordingly.

12 Old Culture
Some activities are demeaning and age-inappropriate for older people

This is a long-held view, that certain activities which are most commonly understood as a feature of childhood – such as using a doll, playing with a ball, reading a picture book, watching a children's television programme

– are inappropriate for use as therapeutic interventions with older people. It is a view which holds that to offer such activities to older people is insulting, and has a potential to encourage them to regress and to act in a childish manner.

New Culture
No activity is, in itself, demeaning or age-inappropriate

We have discussed the idea that no activity is inherently therapeutic – that ultimately therapy lies in a person's own use of an activity to positive effect. We have to apply that principle to the statement above as well. No activity is inherently demeaning, insulting or age-inappropriate; positive or negative effect lies in a person's view of, and response to, that activity. If an older person chooses to engage in an activity such as playing with a doll, with clear evidence of enhanced function and/or well-being, then it is clearly not perceived by that person as demeaning or insulting. You and I might consider it age-inappropriate, but of what consequence is that? We are concerned here with person-centred and person-led care, not with imposing our own values and views upon a person.

Those who work with people who have dementia should also be aware that a return to a preference for increasingly simple, childlike activities is to be expected over the later course of the condition. This is not 'wrong' and should not be discouraged. Indeed, one might argue that for a person operating on increasingly diminished capacities, such activities are entirely age-appropriate. We need to be guided by the person themselves. The rule of thumb with any intervention is to look for the impact. If what we are seeing as a result of our intervention is a person experiencing improved function and increased well-being, we cannot go too far wrong.

13 Old Culture
More research should be aimed at identifying activities which are of special benefit to the older person

It has been pleasing to see the volume of research around therapies increasing over recent years. But research in this area seems currently to be inextricably locked into a time-warp – a rather dangerous notion that borrows from traditional research into physical therapies an assumption that *this* therapy is likely to have *these* benefits with *that* particular group of people. A brief trawl through the volumes of research around reality orientation, reminiscence and (more recently) multi-sensory approaches, will reveal a preponderance of randomised controlled trials (RCT), long deemed the research method of choice for determining the therapeutic benefits of a particular therapy or approach. In fact, all an RCT can do is to tell us that this particular approach helped this group of experimental subjects a lot, that group of subjects not at all, and the rest to varying degrees across the spectrum in between. This is quite extraordinarily unhelpful for the clinician who works with individuals. The field of therapeutic endeavour has shown a marked reluctance to move away from this research model. Until it does, we are not going to advance very significantly in the matter of determining therapeutic efficacy with older people, and raising its profile in the healthcare world.

New Culture
More research should be aimed at identifying that range of activities which are of special benefit to my client, Mrs Clark

It is my personal view that a great deal of research funding has been misdirected when it comes to RCTs and therapy. They are of extraordinarily little value to the clinician whose whole working life revolves around the question 'What specific intervention produces specific changes in a specific individual under specific conditions?'. Research monies should be assisting the clinician to answer that question. The clinician knows that no one therapy or intervention is therapeutic for all, and that any one therapy or intervention will have different effects on different people. It may also have different effects at different times, under different circumstances, in the same person.

To illustrate: the clinician has discovered that the bubble tube in the sensory room seems to have a calming effect on Mrs Clark, who will sit and gaze and stroke it and sometimes doze off in front of it. She has used it to very positive effect on occasions when Mrs Clark has been particularly agitated and restless. But there have been two or three occasions when the bubble tube appears to have had the opposite effect, and alarmed and repelled her. It seems that the clinician has a very useful therapeutic tool in the bubble tube, although if she cannot discover what it is which triggers the alarm, she cannot ethically continue to use it. How is she to find out? This is the kind of question with which most clinicians need assistance. Occasionally answers are readily forthcoming. Sometimes they are not. When they are not, single subject (or system) research methodology comes into its own. Single system methodology enables the clinician to measure the subject against himself, response against response, unlike the RCT in which a subject's responses are measured against those of other subjects.

Single system research can enable the clinician to investigate all kinds of complex clinical questions. The problem is that in the practice setting it is always ongoing and therefore time consuming. The average clinician rarely has the time to apply such rigorous procedures to practice. Nevertheless this is the route to best practice and this is what needs funding.

I started this chapter with Kitwood. It seems fitting also to end with him:

What, then, lies at the core of the difference between the two cultures? I think it is this. The old culture is one of alienation and estrangement. Through it we are distanced from our fellow human beings, deprived of our insight, cut off from our own vitality. The old culture is one of domination, technique, evasion and buck-passing. To enter the new culture is like coming home. We can now draw close to other human beings, accepting all that we genuinely share. (Kitwood, 1995, p11)

'Accepting all that we genuinely share': that for me is the key difference of the new culture. It is a culture which levels hierarchies and demolishes the 'us and them' model of healthcare (they are sick, we will make them better; they are damaged and disturbed, we will set them right; they don't know how to deliver themselves from their distress, we have the answers). One of the great tensions (and conversely one of the great freedoms) of activity provision is that, unlike most other healthcare professions, there are no standard procedures for interventions. It is not possible for any practitioner to say 'This is how you deal with that; this intervention is the correct one for that condition'. In this field there are no fonts of knowledge with all the answers; there are no experts. We are negotiators, facilitators, enablers. Our task is to come alongside our clients and work with them on a basis of equality towards a therapeutic end. The therapeutic relationship is one of mutuality and reciprocity, a sharing of personal resources to an agreed conclusion. This is the new culture of activity provision, earthed in, and generating from, relationship. Only when the healthcare world has fully understood this, will activity provision take its rightful place in the care of older people with a chronic disability.

CHAPTER **2**

The Developing Culture in its Political Context

Rosemary Hurtley

You don't stop doing things because you grow old. You grow old because you stop doing things. (Dame Thora Hird, 2002)

Introduction

It is important to consider the current position of therapeutic activities within the political and demographic context. There are also some considerations that include wider reference to ageism, lifelong learning, best value and the health promotion agenda. The current realities of the experience of the older person in a range of care settings will be highlighted within the context of their subjective quality of life. The roots of the current growth in activity provision in long-term care from an occupational therapy perspective will be outlined in the light of policy-driven changes, with its original emphasis on occupation for health. From this will emerge a picture of future needs and trends. I shall try to gaze into the future in terms of challenges to the current status quo, and suggest some 'blue skies' options for the next generation of more demanding baby boomers and for our own futures.

Background

The use of occupation to promote health for people of all ages has been recognised and practised by the occupational therapy profession since well before the National Health Service (NHS) began. It is based on the science and art of health through occupation, now underpinned by the theories of occupational science. However, occupational therapy in different forms can be traced back even to biblical examples. It is concerned with the activities necessary for life, activity or activity limitation, social participation and lifestyle restriction as they relate to the individual's experiences, needs and aspirations (College of Occupational Therapists, 2002). Due to recent developments, organisational structures and working environments within health and social care have changed. Long-term care of older people has been fragmented across the statutory, voluntary and private sectors. Adequate funding for both quality of life and health needs has not followed. Due to a recognition of need, however, there has been a recent growth in the demand for meaningful occupation for older people who sit around walls 'like a geriatric pageant in death row'. Two-thirds of members of the Relatives and Residents Association are reported to be most concerned about the high boredom levels and lack of purposeful activity. The absence of access to both state registered occupational therapists or other resources led to the introduction of other means of providing 'activities or diversional therapy', and the development of various models of the activities coordinator/organiser. This has been driven from within the sector, by voluntary organisations such as the National Association for Providers of Activities for Older People (NAPA) and Age Concern, commissioners, relatives and even homes wishing to be more competitive in providing for those with chronic illnesses who have traditionally required the support of a long-term caring establishment of one sort or another. The needs and issues raised, however, are equally applicable to older people in sheltered housing and other community settings.

The Context of Social Change

Post-war years have seen an ageing of the population in the industrialised world. People are now living longer and birth rates are in decline. These two factors have resulted in a rapid increase in the percentage of older people, a trend that will continue during the next 20 years. Some of the most relevant social changes affecting welfare over the last 30 years include increasing family breakdown, more women in the workplace and a greater emphasis on, and awareness of, disability rights. There has been a noticeable shift to the nuclear family, due to the ease of geographic mobility, and a loosening of family obligations. There are thus fewer informal carers, in particular middle-aged women who formerly made up a large part of the army of volunteers available in the UK. All these factors have led to an increased need for more formal options for long-term care. Projections suggest that a further 1.3 million places will be needed to cope with an increasing demand for long-term care facilities by 2050 (Telling, 1998).

The Problem

Since political devolution, UK-wide coherency has become increasingly complex between the different developing systems in the separate countries of Britain. The modernisation of health and social care is being prioritised differently in each country. For example, the National Service Framework for Older People (NSF) only applies in England. Therefore the current policy thrust for joint planning and integrated 'whole systems working' is the only way forward to prevent confusion (College of Occupational Therapists 2002).

Over the last hundred years, the long-term care of older people who are without means has moved from its origins in the workhouse to the voluntary hospital, and finally to NHS long-term care provision. This process brought with it, in the first instance, the development of the geriatrician, now referred to as the Consultant in Old Age Medicine. There is more emphasis today on exercise and meaningful occupation for maintaining health and promoting a better quality of life. In my own professional experience working for a health authority during the early 1980s, I supervised occupational therapy helpers who provided full-time activities for patients in a large long-stay hospital. Many of these institutions were adapted from the original workhouse where there were both educational and occupational opportunities as part of the fabric. The meaningfulness and quality of these activities, however, varied across the country, ranging from Dickensian and oppressive goings-on, to a more benign experience (for its day) in different regions. The current picture is one where some of the same client group has now moved out of the NHS into the more fragmented private and voluntary sector, about 70 per cent of which is financed by the state.

Owing to demographic changes and the development of medicine and lifestyle changes, the increase of the very old should be seen as a success. Since records began, only 4 per cent of the population over 65 have required long-term care, but this percentage has now increased at the same time as their numbers have grown. Despite the majority of older people leading more active and independent lives, there has been a commensurate increase in the incidence of chronic illness such as arthritis, stroke, heart disease and dementia. These result in the deterioration of cognitive and/or physical functions, and make increasing demands on the community services. During the 1980s there were perverse financial incentives for local authorities to place older people in residential care earlier than was often necessary. This was due to the legislation of that time, and led to a surfeit of providers who saw quick financial gain from this segment of the population. However, this was to change in the next decade with the Community Care Act 1993 and the closure of many psychiatric hospitals, which served to emphasise the preferred option of caring in the community, meaning, in practice, caring 'by' the community.

It took about 7 years from inception before the full effects of this legislation were realised. We now clearly see a very different type of older person entering long-term care settings. They enter homes much later, present with complex care needs, and cloud the boundaries of admission criteria between residential and nursing care.

Ageism has been inherent in much policy development over the years, with old age depicted as a problem in relation to healthcare, lower income, poor housing, transport and even the paucity of facilities for daily living which we all take for granted. In particular, the approach to long-term care in a range of settings has been seen as the management of decline, rather than a dynamic, positive approach to ensure that older people lead the kind of fulfilling life through which they are still able to contribute to society.

Demography

Evidence presented by the Royal Commission on Long Term Care (Sutherland, 1999) confirms the rise in numbers of the over-65 age group, which is projected to increase by almost 57 per cent between 1995 and 2031. However, the number of over eighty-fives will rise by 79 per cent. By 2050 there will be three times the number of older people than there are today. A younger person today is expected to live to well over 80. This leads to a decrease in the working age population and the alarmist myth of the 'demographic time bomb' (Mullan, 2000). The media speak of our extended old age not as one of the greatest achievements of the twentieth century, but rather as a problem, describing older people stereotypically as 'passive recipients', who make demands on a creaking welfare system in which they are seen to be incapacitated or redundant. It is, however, dependency, rather than old age, that gives rise to the need for care. Although there is a direct link between age and chronic illness, it must be kept in perspective alongside the facts (Richards, 2001):

- only 11 per cent of men and 19 per cent of women over 65 are disabled (1.3 million);
- only 38 per cent of people over 85 are disabled, and a similar percentage are cognitively impaired;
- of 85-year-olds, 80 per cent require some form of help on a daily basis for reasons of physical or mental frailty.

Quality of Life

Research by the Economic and Social Research Council (ESRC, 2001/2) finds that quality of life is generally thought to be an important concept for healthcare delivery in individual patient care. But it is a difficult concept to define and implement, despite the availability of quality of life measuring instruments. It is generally agreed, however, that any of these assessments should essentially report on the individual's subjective viewpoint in a healthcare setting.

There is a general perception that decline always accompanies increasing age. This decline is often associated with social isolation. Some older stroke patients interviewed were able to define quality of life in terms of having the health necessary to participate socially with friends and family, and the ability to get out and about and to have some leisure activities in and outside the home. They also desired sufficient resources to be able to enjoy life. Some defined quality in terms of a broad sense of happiness or enjoyment of life, which invariably included the need for a positive outlook. This research supports previous studies which stated that, while health and functioning (with associated levels of social support, security, safety, independence and adequate finances) are important to older people, there was significant emphasis on the need for sharing in social, educational and local voluntary activities. Recent government initiatives indicate a gradual realisation that access to opportunities for learning may be an integral part of health, well-being and independence in later life (ESRC, 2001/2).

To provide a good quality of life for people with dementia requires specialist training. A report from the Dementia Services Development Centre at the University of Stirling (Chapman & Illesy, 1992) stated that staff are usually better equipped to deal with physical caring needs than emotional and spiritual needs. It recommended an understanding of the importance of stimulation by purposeful activity, thus using remaining abilities. Quality of life is to be promoted, in conjunction with the concern for individuality, dignity, choice and self-esteem. This is taken further, notably in the work by Perrin and May (2000), where issues of well-being and the appropriate use of activities are thoroughly examined for people with dementia.

Issues of Inequality and Ageism

Post-war legislation provided for services to be divided between health and social care. The cultural and bureaucratic differences between the two resulted in difficulties. The emphasis now is on developing a seamless service. Many initiatives promoted the idea of partnership but largely ignored the method of adequate payment for care. One of the greatest anomalies is that those suffering from cancer have received free NHS care, but people with Alzheimer's disease do not. This inequity led to the setting up of the 1999 Royal Commission on Long Term Care. The eventual outcome has resulted in even more complexities, exacerbating inequities and inconsistencies (Richards, 2001). An example of this is the three bands of free nursing care for nursing homes (resulting from the government implementation of the minority report, in preference to the majority recommendation to fund all personal care). This is very difficult to implement, as the procedure is too complex.

Ageism is reflected in the funding arrangements of older and younger people, as evidenced in the allowances set by local authorities for care, which can be nearly 50 per cent higher for the under-65 age group.

Long-term Care in Crisis

Coupled with ageism are the arbitrary anomalies of the criteria set for residential and nursing care arrangements, which appear to have been driven by resources available rather than actual need. Residential homes now care for frailer older people who may be incontinent and often have serious mobility problems or dementia. This has been driven by the reduction in provision of NHS continuing care beds, and the increased need for hospital beds for the acute sector. Means testing also moved many of these people out of the domain of free care. As the post-war nation became owner occupiers, older people were assessed and now pay as they are able, out of capital, not only income. By the 1980s these perverse financial incentives shifted people from hospitals to residential homes where accommodation places grew by 29 per cent between 1981 and 1996 (Richards, 2001). As the long-stay hospitals steadily closed, so the multidisciplinary input, which was the norm (albeit not substantial), was lost. These services, which included occupational therapy, physiotherapy, speech and language therapy and others, had not been costed into the care to be provided by the government-driven, non-statutory sector. During the late 1980s and the 1990s market forces drove homes to work in a competitive environment. The financial opportunism of that time, due to guaranteed government subsidies, encouraged entrepreneurs to set up establishments and drive up fee levels until a benefit ceiling had to be introduced. Between 1993 and 1997 even more nursing homes were developed, as local authorities were to spend 85 per cent of new resources to commission the independent sector. Unfortunately these services have not been set up to match the intended needs-led, choice-driven independence facilitating long-term care. Even more devastating have been the reductions in social services funding. These have led to the provision of only basic levels of care, or what has been described as 'warehousing' of older people, frequently as a result of inadequate staffing.

Sixty thousand beds have been lost in the long-term care sector over the past five years due to the effects of new legislation and other factors. Some of these factors include staff burn-out, high property prices and retirement. Set against the future projection of need, this presents a double-edged standard, where both good and poor caring establishments have suffered on the basis of regulations that emphasise the physical environment over the quality of care. This was eventually addressed by a government U-turn in July 2002, when health secretary Alan Milburn was accused of changing his mind in announcing that the regulations blamed for the closure of care homes would cease to be mandatory. This backtracking of standards, now to be interpreted as guidelines only in an attempt to stabilise the sector, may or may not stem the flow of closures. Some might well argue that the standards should have remained in situ as they were originally implemented to raise the quality of care for the older person. This change of direction might give out the wrong message to home owners, and deter the potential progress in which some homes have already started to invest. It is important to consider some of the history of the sector and discuss other pressures.

The Culture of Change

An attempt was made in the early 1980s to set the standards for residential care by legislation and government directives.

The Registered Homes Act 1984

The inspection methods that derived from this legislation were replaced in 2002 by the National Care Standards Commission (NCSC). Paragraph 12/9 of the Act stated that homes 'should make suitable arrangements for the training, occupation and recreation of residents'. Different health authorities added their own emphases on activity provision for nursing homes that varied across England. For example, one health authority in the south-east of England had guidelines (published in 1984) which stated that residents should:

- have skilled sensitive care to enable them to enjoy the highest possible quality of life;
- be aware of and have access to community and social facilities;
- be able to go out freely and should be allowed to continue interests and hobbies which they had prior to entering the nursing home. For the more able patients, outings and shopping expeditions should be organised.

A Midlands inspectorate recognised in more detail those functioning at different levels, in that even those with 'impaired cognitive ability have been shown to retain more of their abilities when in a stimulating environment, rather than being left to their own devices, to wander without apparent direction, or to sit for long periods with few interactions'. Recreation is described here as 'a broad concept to cover mental, social and emotional involvement in activity, be it passive or active, individual/group, indoor/outdoor, with a range of people, structured/unstructured, spontaneous or planned'. This inspectorate also recommended an individual profile to record interests, social contacts, hobbies and preferences as well as concentration levels.

The Centre for Policy on Ageing

Another influence on the provision of activities in care homes was the publication of the Home Life 2 code of practice by the Centre for Policy on Ageing (CPA, 1996). However, there was only a brief mention of the therapeutic benefits to be derived from being both physically and mentally active, and a suggestion that all homes should be providing stimulation of this sort for their residents. Some examples of activities were outlined, with their likely benefits, but only four lines were devoted to the needs of people with dementia. Owing to some further rather unrealistic recommendations (as perceived within the sector), this document was not taken as seriously as it was intended.

The Human Rights Act 1998

This legislation regulates the activities of all public authorities, including the National Care Standards Commission (NCSC) and local authority homes. Within this Act are Articles 2 (Right to Life), 3 (Inhuman or Degrading Treatment or Punishment), 8 (Respect for Private Family Life, Home and Correspondence) and 9 (Freedom of Thought, Conscience and Religion), as outlined by Cooper (2002). It is conceivable that a lack of provision of activity in care settings could be construed as a source of degrading treatment that may arouse anguish or a sense of inferiority resulting in humiliation or debasement. Similarly a lack of specialist facilities to allow normal family life activities to take place, or a failure to provide access or transport to a place of worship and the practices that surround it, are all likely to discriminate against the well-being of older people.

Modernising Health and Social Services and All Our Futures: The Report of the Better Government for Older People

Published by the Department of Health in 1998 and 2001 respectively, both of these documents encourage the provision of opportunities for exercise as a means to better health and the broadening of social networks.

The Care Standards Act 2000

This Act responded to longstanding criticisms within the care sector relating to inequitable enforcement of the Registered Homes Act 1984 throughout England. Different local authorities appeared to have different priorities, and there was a perception within the private sector that the inspectorate was not independent and could manipulate the system to some extent. In particular, the legislation addressed the issue of the perceived 'unequal playing field' in relation to care home placements, as well as the lack of equality of inspection across all providers of long-term care. The result was a new and independent inspectorate called the National Care Standards Commission, which aimed to bring equality to all service providers. At the time of writing the irony is that this too has changed and moved under the aegis of the Social Services Inspectorate (SSI) to become the Commission for Social Care Inspection (CSCI).

National Service Framework for Older People (NSF)

Issued by the Department of Health in 2001, this is one of the most significant pieces of recent change. The new service standards should be set alongside the National Minimum Standards for care homes and its monitoring by the new National Care Standards Commission. Health and social care are being drawn closer together. All these recent developments have common underlying principles, which are:

   support and promotion of independence;
   social inclusion;
   rights and choices for service users and carers;
   better care and improved standards;
   care at, or close to, home;
   whole spectrum of options;
   integrated across boundary working.

The National Service Framework in particular is about age discrimination, person-centred care, increased choice, prevention and rehabilitation. Standard 8 explicitly is about promoting an active and healthy life to extend healthy life expectancy: 'The health and well-being of older people is promoted through a coordinated programme of action led by the NHS with support from councils.'

The National Minimum Standards support quality services that ensure attention to the whole spectrum of personal healthcare needs and choices, along with a focus on improved quality of life in all care facilities for older people. The health-promoting work of organisations such as the National Association for Providers of Activities for Older People (NAPA) and EXTEND (a charity promoting physical exercise for older people) are of particular significance here.

The Building Capacity and Partnership in Care 2001
This strategic document provides a positive challenge from the government, recommending a greater involvement of the private sector at the planning stage of developing new facilities, as well as in service delivery to form a part of the 'whole systems' working agenda. The aim was to regenerate the sector, looking ahead to try to solve the capacity problem. Nevertheless, in reality it is difficult to implement as the sector is so fragmented. This is a weakness, as it is difficult to change attitudes in a culture that often functions in a modus operandi of crisis management.

Care Homes for Older People: National Minimum Standards
Published in 2001 by the Stationery Office for the Department of Health, this document stated that service users should:

- find the lifestyle experienced in the home matches their expectations and preferences, and satisfies their social, cultural, religious and recreational interests and needs;
- maintain contact with family/friends/representatives and the local community as they wish.

It is also stated that activities must be appropriate to needs and capabilities, people must have more of a say in the social life of the home and more opportunities in/outside the home. In addition, activities must match their expectations and preferences, and satisfy cultural, religious and recreational interests and needs. It is also pointed out that homes are expected to ensure that 'the routines of daily living and activities made available are flexible and varied to suit service users' expectations, preferences and capacities'. Furthermore, interests must be recorded and users should be given opportunities for stimulation through leisure and recreational activities both in and outside the home. Particular emphasis is placed on the importance of activities appropriate for people with dementia, other cognitive impairments and a range of sensory, physical and learning difficulties.

Purposeful activity and occupational well-being are both concepts whose implementation is required to meet government policies and priorities. These include:

- promoting independence, working towards achieving a lifestyle of choice by focusing on both health and social care needs and by preventing avoidable and unwanted dependence;
- social inclusion, with a range of measures to achieve National Service Framework objectives;
- public health and the health promotion agendas, which should incorporate leisure and productivity.

In particular, there is a need to promote healthy and balanced lifestyles as well as to reduce lifestyle restrictions and activity limitation by timely best value interventions (College of Occupational Therapists, 2002). These are refocusing our attention on how care will be delivered in future.

In July 2002 a further consultation document was released, seen as a U-turn on the physical standards originally required and potentially giving the impression of letting home owners 'off the hook' by relaxing the pressure on driving standards upwards within an agreed time frame. This has given mixed messages to providers who have let the sector down in the past by delivering poor standards. They may take comfort and not bother to raise the standards of their facilities. Those more conscientious providers, who have invested enormous amounts of time and money in improvements are likely to feel demoralised and undermined as poorer providers are permitted to continue with inferior provision. However, it is unlikely that the inspectorate will relax their standards on poor delivery of care or a failure to respect the rights of those in their care.

The Lifelong Learning Agenda

Lifelong learning is about continued non-formal learning experiences which maximise growth and personal development. The Fourth Age Carry on Learning initiative by the National Institute of Adult Continuing Education (NIACE) has successfully obtained government funding from 2001 for three years, on the basis that active learners enjoy healthier lifestyles and maintain their independence. The *Fourth Age Learning Report* (Soulsby, 2000) highlighted a universal acceptance that engagement in learning and similar activities can enhance quality of life, lessen dependency and increase well-being. The Department of Health has funded NIACE to develop a programme of learning activities for older people in care settings that will help to overcome barriers and attitudes which negate such consistent provision. This involves collaborative working at all levels with some considerable attention paid to attitude and culture change.

NAPA is also involved in a partnership project, Growing with Age, which develops this topic of lifelong learning opportunities further. It promotes encouraging the resources of voluntary organisations into care homes to widen the range of activities on offer. Designed to improve quality of life, residents are offered greater opportunities to engage with the wider community both within and outside the home, assisting the activities coordinator to provide a richer range of activities.

The Health Promotion Agenda

Attention is being paid increasingly to the area of disease prevention and health promotion for older people (particularly in relation to older people who fall) as set out in the National Service Framework, which aims to promote a more dynamic proactive and integrated approach. This includes the promotion of exercise programmes in a range of settings for older people, due to an increased awareness of the effect that declining functional performance has on health resources (Kelly, 2002). Further research evidence is needed in this area. Nevertheless it is interesting that a 1998 publication from the Royal College of Physicians (RCP), *Enhancing the Health of Older People in Long-Term Care*, emphasised the importance of access to relevant health professionals, in stating the need for positive care for people with dementia and in detecting and managing depression.

Further to this was a significant collaborative report, *The Health and Care of Older People in Care Homes: A Comprehensive Interdisciplinary Approach* (Royal College of Physicians and Royal College of Nursing, 2000). This report emphasised the need for more multidisciplinary input and furthermore recommended the Teaching Nursing Home model with a more research-based approach to improve healthcare outcomes for older people.

It is emphasised that increased resources will be required to maintain health and postpone the disabling effects of chronic disease. In addition to the problem of disease is the care process itself. From this arises problems of over-dependency, a fear of falling and a higher incidence of depression that will frequently result in poor motivation. Kindness-induced dependency serves to increase weakness and enforce disuse. It is encouraging that government policies are beginning to target the provision of exercise facilities both in the community and in care settings. Moreover, it is evident that the introduction of health promotion strategies which empower staff to introduce a broader range of regular activities will help to promote health and improve quality of life.

The Future

Understanding the complex system of funding care home placements is stressful for the client and their families. The complex picture we see today is one where private residents, who have sold their assets to pay for care, are subsidising some of the 70 per cent who are paid for by the state and who are living under the same roof. They receive the same care, but sometimes pay double for it, as owners struggle to meet the costs of increasing regulation and workforce legislation. This has resulted in a driving down of quality provision where a wide choice of activities and fulfilling lifestyles for the older disabled person might have been offered. Another consequence was the concentration of ownership in the sector that accelerated between 1996 and 1997 through a series of mergers and acquisitions. Many small operators closed due to the demands of the National Minimum Standards for care homes for older people, which required them to alter the living environments to meet new guidelines, with no additional financial help. It is likely that this current low concentration of homes will increase considerably, giving rise to the equivalent of supermarket chains of local monopolies. This raises concerns about the quality of services provided, 88 per cent of which are in the independent sector (Holden, 2002).

Research published by the Joseph Rowntree Foundation (Laing, 1998) and more recently by the King's Fund (Henwood, 2002) claimed that there are considerable disparities between fees paid by the state and the true cost of care. A government announcement in July 2002 promised greater investment in the sector, but it remains to be seen what will actually happen.

Age Concern England statistics reveal that two-thirds of the population over 75 are women and have longstanding illness. Dementia affects 20 per cent of those over 80. The chances of living in a care home are 1 per cent for 65 to 74-year-olds; they increase to 5 per cent for the 75 to 84 age group and to 7 per cent for those over 85. Age Concern believes that all older people have the right to expect their later life to be both fulfilling and an enjoyable experience, regardless of their personal circumstances. By 2021 there will be 12 million people over 65, with a corresponding reduction in younger people, and 20 per cent of the population will be retired. By 2030 there will be 35,000 people aged over 100. The Debate of the Age 1998/9 set out to raise awareness about the ageing society and to influence policy relating to demographic ageing. Considerable dissatisfaction with long-term care in the independent sector was highlighted, and this sector provides more health and social care beds than the NHS and local authorities combined. In addition there was a clear desire to promote healthy lifestyles, preventative measures and better training of professionals.

The King's Fund report *Future Imperfect?* (Henwood, 2002) refers to issues of an ageing population and workforce shortages. The tension between containing costs and promoting quality was paramount, along with the patchy development of staff skills and values. Problems with staff recruitment and retention, inconsistent training of care staff and several management deficits were also highlighted in this report. It suggested that a radical change is needed before care work can be elevated in status and value, contrary to the prevailing belief that it is unskilled work which anyone can do. This will require further investment, training and leadership.

The National Director for Older People's Services and the Department of Health aim, by means of the NSF, to root out age discrimination in health and social care and to increase direct involvement of older people and their families in decisions that affect their care. Hopefully this will include all groups of older people, and not simply concentrate on those living in their own homes, as those in long-term care settings are also part of the community. Since the latter group have an increased risk of health deterioration, this will in turn affect the need for acute hospital services. This was highlighted in a recent informal survey for the Department of Health, which discovered that across England about 45 per cent of 'delayed discharges' come from the care home sector.

Projects such as Growing with Age (NAPA), Active for Later Life (British Heart Foundation) and Fourth Age Learning (NIACE) will yield results to demonstrate the benefits of providing a range of meaningful activities using various resources. It is important that others will be added which will demonstrate how, in addition to exercise, well-targeted and meaningful activities can contribute to positive health outcomes. These include the prevention of functional deterioration, the promotion of increased engagement and quality of life experience for the most vulnerable.

The lifelong learning and the social inclusion agendas, along with strategies to promote health, social care and well-being for older people, are the key areas where therapeutic activity needs to prove its worth. We must take pains to point out that a lack of access to health promotion facilities such as exercise and activity programmes will increasingly put at risk the oldest group living in supportive environments.

The occupational therapist values occupation as the means of achieving personal autonomy, self-fulfilment and interdependence across the health and social care divide. It is clear that this profession needs not only to align itself more closely with its original roots, but also to support the work and direct the training and supervision of a much needed but professionally rudderless, group of activity service providers in the field. Occupational therapy is traditionally about developing individual skills, competence and satisfaction in daily living occupations, and not just a 'reductionist' medical approach concerned with basic survival in self-care. The barriers here are not just organisational but attitudinal (College of Occupational Therapists, 2002). The profession needs to define a specific role for itself in this field, working closely with organisations such as NAPA and NIACE. If the performance of activities with purpose and meaning is to promote and maintain health and quality of life, then there needs to be a strategic shift of emphasis. Much can be done to support the army of activities coordinators in the field who are already tackling this issue. As the majority of older people in care settings have chronic health conditions, not only must the occupational perspective be restored, but serious lobbying and advocacy also need to take place in order to enshrine activity provision as central to the process of modern health and social care practice for older people who are now living longer lives.

Different models of care will be needed to meet the wide-ranging and often non-conformist spectrum of tastes, values, experiences and leisure preferences, ranging from abseiling to bingo. This must be accompanied by appropriate staffing levels, training and an inclusion of family contributors to provide real delivery of person-centred activities. Person-centred activity provision is only possible if there is true partnership between staff, residents and their relatives (Eales et al, 2001). It is only then that residents will experience a good 'fit' between their values and preferences. In order to meet the choice-driven demands and future needs of older people in a postmodern age, the government must be concerned with the structure of the market to provide for a variety of tastes and preferences, as much as for the conditions within homes themselves.

Conclusion

I have explored the development of care provision for the frail older members of society against some of the policy background, illustrating the complexities of a fragmented and inequitable provision of long-term care. Within these settings, the importance of meaningful activity and how it fits into the current and future policy agendas has been discussed. It is a provision that can only gain in efficacy, and should be enshrined in daily care practices. Proactive intervention alongside other restorative and enabling interventions require adequate resources to enable older people to wear their age with dignity, rather than as a burden to society. As age is a relative continuum, the challenge must be urgently to debate the level of care and quality of life experience that we would all like to receive if we need them ourselves one day.

CHAPTER 3

The Unit Manager: The Key to Cultural Change

Keena Millar and Sylvie Silver

'**N**O, SHE'S NOT READY. WE'VE BEEN BUSY. It's alright for you swanning around all day talking, but we have to do the real work.' This was delivered at high volume in front of two carers and a resident. As I walked away, the lump in my throat grew, half in anger – I always cry when I'm angry – and half in distress at the look on the resident's face. As Matron walked past she cautiously asked if I was OK. 'Give me ten minutes to walk round the grounds and I'll tell you', was my reply. An hour later we talked through the latest incident, looking yet again at ways to share the belief we both held that our care home's culture needed to change.

We have worked together for seven years in a 40 bed nursing home. We are registered for old age (over 65 years) and up to four terminally ill residents. Set in landscaped grounds on the edge of the Surrey green belt, we cater largely for private income residents. The downside of this lovely setting is attracting staff when public transport is poor and salaries for local house cleaners far outstrip what we can offer. From those early days of no activity provision to our current regular, structured programme, we have trodden a hard road together. As matron and prospective activity organiser we had an immediate rapport at interview. This has grown into a mutual respect for each other's background, knowledge and experience, and has been the foundation for a solid working relationship. These are our accounts of this journey.

The Manager

Thirty years ago I encountered life for the elderly in a medical ward, while training to be a nurse. It was obviously no place to spend the rest of one's days. I knew there had to be more to life than sitting in a chair and looking at your feet all day until you were dead. A strong belief that there is potential in all of us, no matter how old, and no situation which could not be improved, has been the driving force behind my philosophy ever since.

It is an awesome task providing contentment for perfect strangers, but the absolute responsibility for this lies with the home manager who must motivate and encourage all staff to provide a rewarding lifestyle for the residents in their care. Practical steps need to be taken to ensure that staff understand how they can contribute to the process that will provide favourable outcomes in terms of lifelong satisfaction for residents. Staff need to consider what they are actually doing when they look after elderly people in a care home. This is a specialised area of care, equally as specialised as areas such as paediatrics or obstetrics. Midwives would rightly argue that their training is specific to their role, and that they have honed and developed their skills to meet the needs of pregnant women and their babies. Similarly specific skills need to be developed for care of the elderly. General nursing is the personal care people cannot do for themselves. In elderly care the aim is to minimise impairment and maximise ability. Nurse managers in this environment need to be educators, leaders and personal developers. Their role is to 'conduct the orchestra'. Having recognised that the long-term care environment is unique, there are three key areas that a manager needs to consider, all of which are interwoven:

1 The physical environment
2 The philosophy of care
3 The culture of activity provision

Put another way, people's surroundings, how they are treated and how they spend their day, are the keys to sustaining a satisfactory quality of life. Everyone needs to feel comfortable and relaxed in their physical surroundings, to know that they will be treated with dignity and respect and to be offered opportunities to engage in activity. Realistically, the philosophy of care is a concept which all staff in the team need to sign up to and understand in order to achieve the desired effect. A holistic, rounded approach to the way in which we care for residents needs to be guided and led.

Some of our trained nurses were very sceptical about care being anything other than nurse-led and with tangible outcomes. Most of our nurses had trained in the 1960s and 1970s. Training then was rigid and clinically based. Nurses were rarely questioned about the decisions they made. Patients were generally subservient and junior or unqualified staff would not dream of challenging a decision made by a superior. Nor were nurses under much pressure to be accountable. This changed in 1993 when alterations to the Post Registration Education and Practice Project by the Nursing and Midwifery Council required proof of updating knowledge in a chosen field of work over a three-year period. Residents and relatives are now empowered with knowledge not previously held. Care staff are being trained to a higher standard and encouraged to understand what they are doing and why. Trained nurses now have to be confident in their decision making and prepared to defend their decisions at many levels.

Getting someone washed and dressed and administered with the right medication or dressing should never be the sum total of the nurse's role. If a nursing home admits people for the rest of their lives, the service provided must be as diverse as the people it admits. From experience, there tends to be a greater focus on the needs of the very dependent resident who has high medical and nursing needs, and not so much focus on those who can wash and dress themselves but who need attention given to how they will spend their day. No resident should feel abandoned and worthless but should have some purpose in life, some enjoyment, a reason to go on developing and to believe, as someone once said, that you are never too old to learn.

When I became the matron/manager in 1988 there was no real word in nursing terms that I knew of for 'activities'. My first instinct was to get the residents into a context where we could offer social interaction, that is, into the communal sitting room. The problem with this was that nothing looked worse than a group of elderly people sitting in a circle staring at each other in silence. Sight and hearing difficulties made any interaction difficult. Some residents had lived alone for over 20 years. To be put into a large group and expected to talk was at worst frightening, at best uncomfortable. Nursing staff were all so busy dealing with other residents that no one was available to facilitate social interaction. Area health authorities were keen on sitting rooms and communal spaces, but I soon realised that the residents seemed happier in their own rooms with easy access to their own toilet. At that time I concentrated on staff attitudes to enable residents to be themselves and to do what they could for themselves. I wanted staff to rid themselves of the notion that they had to seek permission to engage in anything that was not an obvious 'nursing' action. I wanted a culture for the home that was natural, relaxed, warm and friendly and one that promoted self-esteem.

During this time I was very much directing the day-to-day care as the matron, working as a trained nurse on shifts, giving handover reports and listening to others report. I routinely asked questions about well-being. Did Mrs So and So seem to be unhappy? Why was that? What could we do to change things for her? I usually did the doctors' rounds and would give instructions to staff afterwards as to how a situation should be handled. It was also important to get away from the word 'patient' and to stop reference to people by room number. This sometimes occurred when the nurse call bleeps showed a room number where assistance was required: 'I'm just going to see what number nine wants'. We had people who resided in the home and they were 'residents'. It worries me now to see care standards statements referring to 'service users'; it is impersonal and, in my view, a backward step. By constantly encouraging staff to look at the residents' needs, I hoped to influence the culture towards the residents adopting an active lifestyle.

It was an encouraging, but also sad day, when a registered nurse left to return to her native Manchester with the comment that she really liked what we were trying to do in the home. That was the first time anyone had acknowledged that something tangible was taking place and we were beginning to see a holistic care approach among the staff. If someone wanted to walk by themselves to supper or if someone wanted to pour themselves a drink, then why not? Did it actually matter when people went to bed or got up, as long as they had enough sleep in 24 hours to maintain well-being?

Later on the home was taken over by a small nursing home group. A number of the other homes had a purpose-built activity room and I thought this an excellent idea. There was an activities organiser appointed, usually called an occupational therapist (OT), although these people held no formal qualifications. I visited one of these homes. The OT room was open to residents mornings and afternoons. Coffee was served and usually some knitting and sewing were available; sometimes guest speakers came along. It was like a Women's Institute meeting.

The new owners were anxious to provide activities in my home. I decided to use one of the large sitting rooms in the home and made it the dedicated area for activities. Most people called it OT. I advertised for an OT person and a part-time lady started who put on knitting and sewing parties and craft events. It felt like a poorly supported club that no one wanted to belong to. Yes, there were now things to do, but who actually wanted to do them? Relatives were happy to see the service, but I realised that the residents, bar a few, were not anxious to attend. Sight problems and arthritic hands simply showed up what people could no longer do. I felt that craft activities were not the answer as a communal event. These could easily be done by those who were keen and able in their own rooms if they wanted to.

Over a three-year period we had three OT ladies in post. The advertisements composed by the then owners of the home brought forward applicants who were keen 'to do things'. There was great disappointment when residents did not want to take part. The majority of staff were not encouraging residents to attend in a positive way. It was perceived as just more hard work to take a resident to an activity session. They were also scathing of the OT person's workload if she spent all day with just one person in the OT room. Two of these ladies had previously been carers and seemed to have the right attitude towards the residents. However, they had no skills in setting up and running group activities, and no training was available. They also had to contend with their colleagues believing they were skiving if they declined to take someone to the toilet while they were busy trying to make Christmas cards. One lady achieved a degree of success when we established a daily routine of taking some residents directly to an activity session from the dining room at lunchtime. I also allocated a carer to work with her each time. It was still largely craft-based activities that were offered, with limited appeal it seemed, but a few friendships developed between residents as a result. Unfortunately family circumstances caused her to leave, and her successors failed to bring the same enthusiasm to the role.

At about the same time, a registered nurse (RN) and I undertook the English National Board 298 course, one module of which was the Biographical Approach to the Elderly. This cemented my original commitment to holistic care and to enabling a resident to have a life beyond getting dressed or having a suppository. Biography work not only looks at past events and achievements, but also at attitudes to life, coping strategies and personhood. We started to look at what made the person now in our care tick, and how we could build and develop on that. Activity provision was clearly going to be important, but most of the staff had seen activities as a hassle and the job of the OT as money for nothing. There was no concept among the trained nurses that activities could be part of a care package. The people who applied for the OT post did not have a broad enough outlook on what might be possible, or any experience in facilitating development or identifying potential. We needed someone who understood the concepts of choice, respect and dignity, and who could base a programme on the needs, likes and wishes of the individuals in our home.

I set about writing a job advert without resorting to the company standard or referring to the expected job description. With the RN from my biography course, I discussed what activity provision we wanted. We agreed that the home needed someone who was friendly, warm and caring; someone who could engage the residents in conversation, build up trust and generate a feeling of *wanting* to be involved in a programme of events. We were delighted to be in a position of choice when we interviewed five applicants for the post.

The Activities Organiser

The advert for this role caught my eye. It was looking for someone to work with elderly people in a nursing home, but the key words that struck me were caring, warmth and conversation. Having spent the previous five years as the manager of a community-based day service for adults with learning disabilities, I was ready for a change and had developed an interest in elderly care. I had experience of preparing individual activity programmes as well as running group sessions, I had trained my own staff team and, more importantly in hindsight, had previously worked as a nursing auxiliary. Matron's phone call offering the post was hesitant on her part, as she knew I was being offered a 50 per cent pay cut. Nonetheless I accepted the challenge of becoming an activities organiser, as I was then called.

On appointment to the nursing home, I was thrown back in time to my hospital days. The uniforms had not changed much, and the day seemed to be dictated by medicine rounds and bathing. My base was to be a large room known as OT where no one seemed to go. My predecessor had left some months before, so I was given free rein to develop the activities culture for the home.

At that time all but two residents routinely stayed in their rooms apart from lunchtime in the dining room, when about 20 people would sit and dine. Next door, in the attractive small dining-room, five residents with high dependency needs were fed by carers. A few residents ventured independently onto the terrace to take some fresh air.

Occasionally a carer would appear and ask if she could bring in a resident who shared a bedroom, and was driving her roommate to distraction. I also appeared to have sole responsibility for a lovely chap who came two days a week for respite care to have a bath and give his wife a rest.

Initially Matron was my sole point of contact. We clearly shared a philosophy of person-centred care and a need to base any activity programme on what the residents wanted. It was obvious that we needed a way of asking residents, both individually and collectively, what they wanted, but most had grown used to a life centred on their bedrooms and were not likely to participate willingly in group activities straightaway. The nursing staff were also used to this gentle pattern of life where they were in control of the day's progress and the residents' whereabouts.

We agreed that I would slowly get to know the residents on a one-to-one basis by visiting them in their rooms and building a relationship of trust. This threw up the first problem. Whenever I was out of OT, particularly on a day when the respite man was in, I would be chased by a nurse or carer and asked why I was not with him. My predecessors had always stayed with him in the OT room, along with the two ladies who liked to come down and paint or do craft. Matron and I would patiently explain to the staff that my role was not going to be room-based, and that everyone was responsible for people in the house, whatever room they were in. We had agreed that I would need to get into residents' bedrooms and get to know them as individuals, building trust and meeting needs, no matter how small. I would often take a resident for a walk in the grounds or adjust their television so that they could see it better. The staff were not used to this approach and were clearly uncomfortable with my apparent autonomy. Rumours came back to me that I seemed to sit and talk all day. Whenever possible I would explain what I was doing and why, but staff were often defensive and assumed I was criticising them for not doing what they should. I soon learnt that I would have to be fairly thick-skinned and not take these comments to heart, although I found it hard.

At one of our regular supervision sessions Matron made a key decision to change the name of the room. It was not an occupational therapy room and I was not an OT. The residents seemed to perceive it as somewhere to avoid at all costs, unless visiting the hairdresser there. It needed a friendlier title, so we decided on The Conservatory, which described it very well. If anyone called it OT I simply did not respond, neither did Matron.

After six months in post I felt confident enough to do a formal survey of the residents. Matron asked me to present the outcome to the whole house staff meeting. I chose a very visual form of graphs to show that the most preferred activity, by a long way, was 'a good conversation', which I had listed along with bridge and sherry parties as possible options. Our next task was to convince the staff that they were well placed to make conversation with residents and that it would be a valid way to spend their time. We have had great success latterly in this area, but are still working to break through the barrier that says it is more important to sort the laundry trolley than to talk to residents.

It was not long before Matron suggested changing my job title. We wanted to convey a message that the role of activities organiser did not mean that the provision of activities was exclusive to the organiser, but that everyone on the staff had a part to play. The title 'Leisure Services Manager' was adopted for several reasons:

1 It strengthened the position. The clear message was that the new title recognised responsibilities for all staff to deliver activities, and that I would 'manage' that delivery across all staff.
2 It broadened the scope of the role to encompass all leisure pursuits which crossed departmental boundaries, such as the provision of televisions and radios.
3 In our setting residents seemed to prefer this description, as most did not want to feel they were 'being organised'.

Initially I had set up small groups of three or four residents who were invited to tea with me. I chose the guests carefully, using biographical information. I sent out attractive handwritten invitations that specified the venue and the start and finish time. I enlisted the chef's help in providing some special cakes, and served everything on bone china crockery purchased from the local charity shop. A vase of flowers and lace cloth completed the setting. I would personally get the residents from their rooms to the appropriate sitting room or table on the terrace.

Once a few friendships had been formed, it was not too difficult to get a group of eight to ten residents together for a sherry and crossword party. This became an established session two mornings a week. Now that we had residents wanting to attend an activity, the next hurdle was to ensure they arrived on time with glasses and hearing aids in place, ready to enjoy a social but challenging activity. Our staff were getting used to the idea that residents could choose, within reason, what time they wanted to have breakfast and to get up and dressed. Now they also had to take into account which residents wanted to attend a function at 11.15. This proved to be a real challenge. We tried endless different systems and methods to get the staff to prioritise their work to meet these appointment times.

The trained nurses in particular felt very pressurised as Matron expected them to ensure that everyone was ready. Some of the staff were beginning to see the value of activities and the benefit to residents and were actively encouraging residents to attend, but a few still believed that, by encouraging independence, the residents had become more vocal and demanding, which made their job harder.

By now I was well-established as part of the management team. All heads of department were accorded equal status by Matron and, although my department was only staffed by me and two cats, I was treated as a manager in every sense (only my salary has never reflected this!). My greatest difficulty at this time was the clear chasm that existed between myself and the trained nurses. I was finding it hard to be accepted as someone who had a contribution to make to a resident's well-being. It seemed that what I provided was a nice extra – if it could be fitted in. As a result of one of our supervision sessions, Matron decided I should have regular meetings with the deputy matron, who was head of nursing care. These often threw up more problems than they solved. A major bone of contention was my desire to know about any changes affecting a resident. If someone was ill or had changed medication, it often had a bearing on how they behaved within group activities and how they responded to me during room visits. At that time, few of the trained staff believed I had a need to know. I was not perceived as an equal, had no formal qualifications, and was never invited to offer an opinion. The deputy matron had many problems to resolve and I was not high on the priority list. Matron regularly addressed these issues in trained nurse meetings.

This scenario turned a corner when Matron was asked in one of these meetings whether the trained nurses had to do what the Leisure Services Manager said. Her measured reply was 'Yes', followed by 'It would be wise to listen as her wealth of experience and knowledge of the residents contribute greatly to the residents' well-being and quality of life'.

Slowly the culture began to change as trust was built up on both sides. I tried hard to understand the nurses' and carers' viewpoints, and encouraged them to ask questions of me at any time. I asked endless questions to broaden my knowledge of medical conditions affecting older people. I offered my views on residents' needs, often unsolicited, but now they were accepted as valid and often acted upon.

A major milestone was preparing and delivering a series of training sessions along with one of the trained nurses and a carer who shared our fledgling new philosophy. This trained nurse had become a chronically ill patient herself, and now sympathised with the residents' views on loss of dignity. She was a very lively and strong character who did not shy away from expressing her opinions. We got on well and she did a great deal to convey to other trained nurses what I was trying to do. Her illness was terminal and one of her parting gestures was activity-led. She bought two kittens for the home which have brought endless pleasure to staff and residents ever since.

For the training session she wrote a piece on dignity and staff awareness, and the carer and I prepared role-play sessions on approaching feeding, hearing and sight impairment with dignity and respect. Matron ensured that everyone attended by adjusting work schedules to allow all staff to be present over a number of weeks. Afterwards there was a noticeable increase in the number of staff who would wander into my room for a chat. I was now beginning to feel less isolated and more part of the team. We were also developing our new culture through reflective practice sessions that Matron ran and invited me to contribute to. This helped the carers to see that I could offer activity-based options to ease some of the problems the residents suffered, and help them to address these issues day to day.

My peer group was the heads of department team. We would meet every month and discuss issues affecting each department. This broadened my knowledge and gave me an opportunity to explain what I was doing and why. I also worked alongside other department heads on preparing presentations and implementing the new company quality assurance programme. The department heads usually got together over lunch so we came to know and like each other quite well. They were always particularly supportive of large-scale functions, which meant working closely together and their enthusiasm carried many other staff along with them. Although a grand Christmas meal in Edwardian costumes was hard work, it brought together residents, relatives and staff in a way not previously achieved. Everyone saw each other in a new light and the buzz gained from a team working well together had an impact on morale that lasted some while. Matron always embraced my 'grand ideas' for social functions and actively supported them.

Our long-term plan had been to establish a group session every morning and afternoon with a diverse but regular programme to appeal to most residents. This puts an extraordinary pressure on all nursing staff to get specific people to a given venue by a fixed time. It is not always achievable, but the difference now is that trained nurses and carers alike will stop me in the corridor to explain why someone might be late or that they have been unwell overnight. It is not just the nursing staff who have embraced activities. Matron expects and encourages everyone to be involved. The housekeeping staff lay out the sitting room each day to an agreed plan. The gardener runs a club in the spring and the maintenance man often brings his dog to work. The chef attends a supper social each month to get feedback from the residents and the receptionist sings in the choir.

I have, on occasions, been a thorn in the side of the deputy matron who struggled to share our message with her team. I know that at times

Matron has been pulled two ways by our conflicting demands, but we all shared a common desire to achieve the best we could for our residents. The deputy matron and I now work closely together, from the day she assesses a new resident, to jointly agreeing on an activities package.

A perfect example of our teamwork was a recent discussion of a resident's needs. This lady has been a resident for some years and through chronic illness and recent bereavement had become 'room bound'. Her nursing needs were high, involving gastrostomy feeds and frequent turns. The feed was almost continuous and she had become trapped in her room. We were both concerned about her mental health and sensory deprivation. Together we devised a goal plan. She made calls to the consultant and dietician to get the feed times altered, and liaised with the physiotherapist. I ensured her wheelchair was serviced and suitably cushioned, and that space was available at the sherry party. I prepared the friends she had among the residents about what to expect when they saw her. The hairdresser was asked to come in specially to redo her perm. On the given day, a trained nurse and two carers took their time to get her up, dressed and into the chair. The deputy matron wheeled her along to the sherry party and her friends were delighted to see her. The beaming smile and kisses she blew in response all made the effort worthwhile. She is now regularly coming to three sessions a week and, although she gets tired, her well-being is markedly improved. Her family are delighted at how responsive she now is to their visits. Just as important is the fact that all the staff acknowledge this as a necessity, not a nicety.

Six years on, having established our core programme, we have changed my agenda to looking more closely at how we meet individual needs. It has become accepted practice in the home for staff to pass on residents' wishes and needs to me. This can be viewed two ways. On the positive side, it is good that staff are recognising the importance of Mary getting out for a walk or Fred needing to socialise more. On the other hand, we need to encourage staff to meet these needs themselves within the everyday pattern of care, and not to assume that it is the sole preserve of activities staff. We have established a new care planning process, in line with the Care Standards Commission guidelines. This will allow for greater consultation between key nurses and activities providers which we hope will further develop the new culture. The Care Standards Commission inspectors are tasked with looking at great depth into all aspects of care, including activities provision. All trained nurses and activity staff will have to work more closely together if we are to meet the requirements effectively.

The Manager

Yes, it is seven years since we first re-examined the activity provision in the home, and since our joint undertaking to provide an activity programme to meet the needs of our residents started. Our own past experiences and person-centred philosophy shaped the vision for a quality, active lifestyle for our residents. It has at times felt like an uphill task, yet it is often only when you take a retrospective view across the years that the extent of the change truly becomes clear. Without question, a very great deal has been achieved, yet in many respects I feel we are only at the end of the beginning.

Changing a culture is essentially about changing the attitudes of the people making up the team, changing the vision of each member of a unit team until that team is truly working in harmony towards a common end. In retrospect I understand that it is never easily nor quickly achieved. We have certainly come a long way, but we have yet much further to go.

We have tried in this chapter to describe a little of our journey towards establishing an active lifestyle in our home. But it may be that there are other managers reading this who are at an earlier stage of the journey, so I have tried to pull out what I feel are the key factors in introducing a new culture of activity in a care home. Without question my task would have been extremely difficult without a skilled and experienced activity organiser alongside who has had the staying power to ride out the difficult times. Nevertheless the initiative has had to come from me and the responsibility remains with me. I would want to say to any manager who might be embarking on a similar journey that ultimately you are the key to cultural change in your home. Drawing on the lessons I have learned over these years, I would want to say to any manager wanting to overhaul the activity culture in his or her home that the following provisions will need to be made:

1 You must be committed to person-centred care.
2 You must understand the value of activities.
3 You must be able to explain the value of activities to staff.
4 You must lead by example and show an interest in all events.
5 You must encourage all staff to be involved in activities.
6 You must give an activity organiser frequent, regular supervision.
7 You must commit to training and updating knowledge for activity staff.
8 You must include the value of activities within induction training.
9 You must establish the right environment for the residents.
10 You must provide adequate financial resources for functions, equipment and materials.
11 You must be committed to developing the potential that may arise from any situation or event.
12 You must accept that activity provision is about more than group sessions; that it involves one-to-one work as well as bringing the community into the home.

CHAPTER 4

The Unit Manager: Creating a Positive Influence

Paul Smith

I IMAGINE THAT YOU WILL NO DOUBT have heard about Pavlov and his famous salivating dog (Pavlov, 1928). But are you also aware of some of the other experiments carried out by the early behaviourist pioneers in the name of research: experiments such as passing an electric shock, again and again, through a restrained horse to find out its ultimate response? Although this type of experiment now appears quite barbaric and would not even be granted research approval in our enlightened times, it is from this historic field of work that a number of important theories were formed concerning human behaviour. One in particular, that of 'learned helplessness', might help us to understand the vital importance of occupation as a 'life-preserving essential' in modern care establishments. The details of the horse's ultimate responses are extremely important when viewed in respect of the need we have as human beings to be able (or at least to feel as if we are able) to influence our own present and future circumstances.

We will return to the details of that experiment later when we explore learned helplessness in the context of this work and I hope, as we do so, that the importance of the perception of its influence will become apparent. This theme of helplessness was constantly running through my mind as I prepared to contribute to this much-needed book. I approached this chapter from a number of different writing styles; I tried the counselling, the adversarial, the pleading and the preaching. As one idea superseded another, it became apparent that to project forwards and offer guidance and perhaps even hope through this chapter, to both employees and managers alike, I had simply to look backwards and reflect honestly on how I learned to become a change agent. I realised that by performing this introspection and revealing the results (the things that had not worked as well as the things that did) I might be able to save you a lot of time and some of the heartache I have gone through in my quest for successful outcomes. I hope that if I just give you an honest account of how, in my opinion, the manager makes the final difference – for good or bad – in the modern care establishment, with a particular reference to activity provision, you might find this useful.

Like you, I have been on the receiving end of both good and bad management decisions and strategies as I worked my way through the minefield of the modern NHS and independent sector to my current position as regional manager and dementia nurse specialist. Like you, I have made some good and bad management decisions along the way. I have formed lasting impressions of individuals and their personal styles from the results of these good and bad management practices. While it is true that the pain of bad management practice inflicted upon you can force you to grow as a person, these negative influences can be controlled and directed. The influence we all have on each other should be considered and professional, but we know that this is not always the case.

I created my core style from deliberate self-exploration and informed choice. I ingested a belief system to apply to my management; it is a belief system that can be learned. Good management, I firmly believe, is about mastery of the self, not others. I will try and explain this Zen-like statement as we progress.

In this chapter I will illustrate why care services can be so much better and so much more alive with good activity provision, and why persons in care (and care establishments themselves) can blossom when occupation really means everyone being committed towards a shared purpose. I will show how applying the same quality-related work ethic I have learned will lead to positive influence, which for me has created award-winning teams and satisfied customers across a number of care establishments and care disciplines. It is a method of influence that has been learnt by thousands of others before me.

First, we must understand that there are no longer any easy rides in the care industry and particularly in care homes that provide specialist care such as dementia or rehabilitation. Gone are the days when second-rate qualified nurses and the least able of staff could hide away in poor standard nursing or residential homes (RCN, 1992). The care homes of the present, and especially those of the future, will need to strive to become vibrant and effective providers of excellence in order to survive, as service demand focuses increasingly on value for money and consumer satisfaction. The staff who work in these units will be forced by Standard 30 (relating to education and training) of the new Care Standards Act to become highly skilled and effective practitioners, constantly training and updating their knowledge and practice (Department of Health, 2000). The Royal College of Nursing recognised as long as ten years ago that some of the best minds and most able care practitioners were choosing to migrate into care homes, and this trend seems set to continue (Nazarko, 2002). As a regional manager I believe it is my job to inspire and create a positive influence for these new-style practitioners. The first basic tenet of every team I work within is that the focus of these new services should, above anything else, be consumer-driven and customer led. In our field of caring this translates to the idiom that the needs, wants and desires of the patient, client or resident and their families must dictate our service. (The term 'resident' will be used throughout this chapter to describe the person living in a residential setting.)

I believe that all good care establishments of the future will understand the basic right of the resident to stimulation, occupation and fun. I would like to see that understanding in operation now, and for this basic right to be held up as a benchmark for the industry. When I look for a place in the care homes of the future for a loved one or for myself, the first thing I would want to know is what I or they would be going to do all day. I do not expect the answer to be bingo.

So I ask the question: 'How do we get these services of tomorrow today?' – services that must offer change, challenge, diversity, choice and ultimately results? It is the manager who must take this responsibility and it is only an achievable goal when the manager accepts that he or she is accountable to the staff, the service user and the service purchaser. In essence the manager is a provider – there to serve.

I would like to make an admission. During my time as a manager I have joined every management fad going (except the Ricky Gervais school of office management). I have scientifically managed, strategically managed and used quality, continuous improvement and excellence stratagems. I have looked upon my organisations as living brains, and benchmarked and audited with the best of them. I have upward managed, downward managed and even managed in circles. Am I embarrassed to admit this exotic flirtation with so many differing management styles? Not on your life. If some of the greatest leaders in the last 100 years thought of each of these ideas as the next big thing, who am I to discount them without at least first having a go? I'll tell you something about this rather eccentric and schizophrenic tendency – it has worked wonders for the people I have had the privilege to lead and it also seems to have helped them provide excellent care for the persons in their charge. But how and why should this be? How could flitting about and constantly changing styles and approaches be a good thing, and can we learn anything from it? When reading this, I am sure many people would accuse me of being a jack of all trades and master of none. Of course perhaps they could be right, but first let us examine the evidence.

When I was training in psychotherapy and clinical hypnosis I came across a statement from the father of modern clinical hypnosis, Milton H Erickson. It went something like this: 'Do not try to fit the patient to the theory; rather, if the theory does not fit, create a new one. Create a new theory for each patient' (Bandler & Grinder, 1979). Everyone is different and unique. What is important is what works. Let me repeat that it is not so much what you do that is important, it is whether what you are doing works or not.

Erickson knew that being bogged down in professional dogma or worrying what others thought about his methods did not help those who came to him seeking help. He went on to develop his practice to the point where his innovative and effective treatments became the stuff of legend. If Erickson knew that the secret of high percentage success was diversity, why have thousands of managers (and therapists) persisted with the outdated assumption that one model and one method will work for everyone and in every situation?

One of the reasons why many excellent management strategies are overtaken by the new (which in truth are often only a rehash of even older techniques) is that no one thing works for everything forever. If something is not working in one situation any more, it may simply be stuck or stale. Starting over, perhaps by removing the blockage and changing things just a little, a forward momentum can again be achieved. It is the little slice of change that is needed to start it on the path that is the essential ingredient.

By learning and experiencing many different styles, I have been able to pull out certain techniques or elements of models to deal with varied situations on a day-to-day basis. Some of the old ways still work when aided by a little input from the new. Try not to become imprisoned within the strict confines and boundaries of a set method. A preference for eclecticism fits perfectly with modern care practice where boundaries are being pushed back on a daily basis. In my particular field, dementia care, the best minds are joining the movement now, just as they did in the 1960s and 1970s within the field of schizophrenia. They can feel the energy and drive of those already committed to our cause. Activity provision must also attract these minds, and it is by offering diversity, challenge and rewards that they will come.

In dementia care, because every person is an individual even when they share the same probable diagnosis, working to one model or one style just will not fit any more (if it ever did); it is not accepted and it is obsolete. To work in any field of care these days you have to know how to adapt to interdisciplinary situations, or at least be able to work with someone who complements your own arsenal. Why should management of the care environment be any different? Managers in care are no different. We have to be daring and challenging. We have to push back the boundaries on practice and work with unique staff and create unique teams. We have to shake the status quo, making up new rules as we go.

To me the care profession is so very exciting, and one of the areas least exploited for excitement at the moment appears to be the provision of inclusive activity services. So we should make this the next exciting area for exploration and innovation. Hopefully you are reading this book because you want to make changes – lasting, effective changes. You are aware that something is not happening in your work systems just now, and you want to move it on. I am going to offer some thoughts on how to do that, but as we get started and apply some of these principles I pose three questions:

1 If you are a manager, what have you done in the last six months to ensure that every single one of your employees believes in your vision for activity provision? (Have you a vision?)

2 When was the last time you (or those responsible to you) sat down with each and every employee and asked 'What can we do for you?' If you are an employee, when did you last say the same to your manager?

3 When did you last implement activity-related changes (or indeed any changes) suggested by a resident, a relative or your team?

If you have not done any of these, the following may be difficult reading.

A Positive Approach to Change and Growth in Activity Services

People in care homes keep on growing and developing when provided with the opportunity for activity. I have absolutely no doubt of this because I have personally witnessed it time and time again. Professor Tom Kitwood coined a term in dementia care that is used to describe a condition in which people who have lost abilities through social or care regime deficits regain some of their unused ability once the deficit has been made good. He referred to this as 're-mentia' (Kitwood, 1997). We can see some of this wisdom in the person who comes from being socially neglected or regains some health after illness. But I am referring here to a broader human potential that being involved, engaged and active 'reassembles' within a person who feels forgotten, abandoned or finished, as do many older people coming into care (Wilkinson, 1998). I have personally witnessed individuals blossom and groups of people unite under good activity provision (or, I should say, good inclusive overall care with occupation at its core). I have seen groups of people form lasting, cohesive and supportive social units when occupational needs were addressed in a personalised, but systematic manner.

I have also seen the effect that a lack of thoughtful activity provision has on people, and I have had to intervene in the aggression, disintegration and sense of abandonment this type of care regime produces in both residents and staff (Barker & Davidson, 1998). In fact many people actively construct their own withdrawal from this type of uncaring 'care' as a form of self-defence against the boredom, frustration and prejudice they encounter.

It is not natural to live with a constantly changing group of others who often cannot form lasting or interactive relationships. Neither is it natural to spend all day in the same room trying desperately to act normally, so that these others do not see the 'new you' that is relentlessly emerging from within your illness; the 'new you' that is taking over from the 'old you' that both you and others had grown familiar with; the one that used to make mistakes without being observed, the one who used to be involved and have friends and feel useful; the one who had a family and a social life, and made their own decisions about what to eat and when to get up or go to bed; the one who had money in their pocket, and would not have been seen dead living in a place like this where nothing happens and no one cares and everyone is old except for the carers who are nice, but always too busy to talk. It is not just a condition like dementia that can take away the 'self', but also uncaring, thoughtless and soulless care regimes.

The theory of 'learned helplessness' alluded to earlier may help us to understand a little of a person's reaction to abandonment, boredom and lack of influence. In the behaviourist trials, after trying to escape, fight and retreat, all to no avail, the horse eventually decided simply to endure the shocks. It resigned itself to being unable to influence what was happening to it and just stood and took it (Shenk, 2002). The same has been reported in times of stress, such as war, prison camps, prison and, yes, even in long-term care (Boyce, 2001; Lazarus 1998). When it appears that no amount of asking, fighting, wandering, shouting or pleading changes anything, then people learn to become helpless. They sit and wait for release. Learned helplessness is probably a lot more commonplace than we care to admit, and it is prevalent in modern care establishments.

I was once asked to manage such a place. It had a terrible reputation, it smelt and the staff and residents fought constantly. There was a lack of pride and a lack of principled leadership. In short, the home had been managed not led (I believe that there is a vast difference between management and leadership). The first thing I did was to meet with all staff and begin a process of negotiation. Together we performed a complete system analysis – everything from physical structures through to personal attitudes, and we agreed a plan to change (change is always movement). I presented my vision of what the service could be like, and I embellished this vision with as many positives as possible, to make it compelling both to my audience and to myself. Then we agreed to tackle the largest problems first.

We were unstoppable in the quest to tackle these larger problems. We changed all the staff shift systems and created an activity coordinator post which allowed a much greater focus on the residents' needs. This took some negotiating, but the vision of what would be possible if we did this was so compelling that in the end everyone voted for it. We created new tiers of junior management to allow responsibility and accountability to staff members. We created and invested in training programmes, many of which I performed personally; although I could have given this role away, I wanted to enforce the vision by personal delivery. At every step along the way I asked for feedback. I drew up questionnaires and opinion polls, created suggestion boxes (with small prizes), and answered every group survey with a personal written reply. I graphed these results and showed them against the last month's or last week's results. I set team performance targets, and I created a home mission statement based on principled care delivery and customer satisfaction. At every opportunity we revisited this whole process and rechecked our goals, skills and where we could expand the vision. We did not stop changing, and within a matter of months the home began to be recognised for its excellence and improvements – within one year it was winning awards.

Change towards the new futures suggested elsewhere within this book is an opportunity to grow, to be challenged and to challenge, and adds variety and meaning to our jobs. Anything short of changing our current practices will lead to further frustration, stagnation and complacency and, for some in our care, no change means no hope. They will learn to become helpless.

Why Managers are Good and Bad

I stated earlier that the key person in the creation and maintenance of a good inclusive activity care system is the home manager. Why should the home manager have such an impact on the quality of the provision of an activity programme? Surely the person responsible is the activity provider? Surely the activity provider is the key to the successful implementation of the ideas expounded throughout this volume? You would be quite naive and innocent to think so. Here are the facts in stark black and white. If the home manager does not believe in a structured and eventful day for the residents and staff, and believes that it is better for everything and everyone to be tidy and in their place, then that is just what you will get. Let this last statement act as a warning for any manager reading this chapter. If you do not make your work and living environments vibrant and full of expectation and movement, you will lose your best staff. You will attract the wrong staff and you may damage beyond repair those in your care. Managers must change themselves, but some will not.

To illustrate this warning I will give you a story from my own experience. I was sitting on a national committee that was concerned with creating a systematic approach to the provision of activity programmes over a large number of care environments. On this committee were a number of differing levels of authority and skill, and among our number were activity coordinators. One in particular showed a huge level of skill, enthusiasm and personal belief in the provision of activities, or at least she did at the beginning of our work together. By the time the committee dissolved, this woman was ready to leave the company. It was not the company that was holding her back; as a matter of fact the company was showing itself more than willing to provide both direction and finance in an attempt to change the inherent culture of disorganised activity provision. It was down to the effects of her individual manager.

These in-house dynamics often remain hidden from those further up the ladder (the manager's manager); especially when they forget to talk to junior staff members and rely only on the evidence presented to them secondhand, often from the home managers themselves. The problems this coordinator encountered included favouritism, lack of understanding of dementia, poor support systems, indifference to her suggested approaches and the continuation of a care regime that was task-led and nurse-directed. No matter what initiatives this lady presented, they were not acted upon, or, worse still, other staff were allowed actively to resist them. When she took her continued frustrations to her manager she said that initially she felt the manager had listened, but no action followed. In short, her battle was lost before it began.

This was not a naive member of staff whose emotions ruled her heart. This was a mature and professional woman who found the love of her calling smothered within her. How many others have given way like this to the will of the person in charge? How many of you are those managers? Have you lost the good seed because it fell on stony ground? As much as I have been involved in supporting people like the lady in the example, I often find that attitudes are set out on both sides of the fence. Change is a two-way process, but in an unequal power distribution the stronger of the two forces, the manager, must be prepared to bend the furthest.

Communication is one key, knowledge is another, but the major drive in creating change is belief. This is why change works for good or for bad. If a manager has no belief in the power of occupation as an effective medium in care, then no amount of persuasion from a junior staff member or a senior board member is going to make the slightest difference. Because the manager holds the power, things will not change for the better. For managers truly to believe in activity provision, they need to understand the critical therapeutic benefits for both residents and staff that inclusive activity provision brings.

The Mutual Benefits of Creating a Culture of Inclusiveness and Occupation

There is something very dead about walking into a care home where the prevailing culture is that of task orientation. It can often be seen immediately, and it flows from the manager down, since culture flows from the top down (Gower, 1998). Speaking from my own observations, in these regimes the manager is not usually well versed in the requirements of the shop-floor. There is an aloofness in relationships between staff and, often in stark contrast, there is an over-closeness among certain 'cliques' (just ask the majority of staff and they will tell you of whom this clique consists). There will be a tendency towards an unlived and unused appearance in the environment; or again, in contrast, the appearance can be that of a 'just could not care less' disorder. Care staff never seem to be around, or when they are around they always seem to be busy with anything other than communication. Just watching these staff is a lesson in avoidance. How can anyone walk between groups of communication-hungry people and only talk meaningfully with their opposite peer group care number? It has always amazed me. In a culture of task orientation the residents become like ornaments, or worse like inanimate pieces of furniture – something to be moved or worked around, tidied and cleared away, but never really engaged with.

A culture where the staff are emotionally involved is, by contrast, not always the tidiest, and does not always appear the busiest, but it is by far the hardest to achieve. It is very hard work and it is not for everyone. For good and caring managers this can be a painful realisation. You may have to lose some people because this type of caring just does not suit everyone. You will probably really like some of these staff, and they will usually be very good at other things like organisation and planning; losing these people will have personal and financial implications. Some really great people are very good at nursing, but just not very good at caring.

Good staff however should cost you both emotionally and financially. First, you should pay good people more, but you also have to invest more in them emotionally. Staff know when you really care and when you simply do not. Being principled in leadership means caring for all in your charge. At the end of the day good leadership is about producing effective teams, and a team is only as strong as its weakest link. But if you are the manager, take a long hard look at how you are running your home. Are you the weakest link? Think about it. Are you really investing more in your staff than just an hourly rate? When people are on low wages, the hourly rate is often equated with their sense of being valued. If the rate is not high, something else must be around to keep them. Everyone must be on board together, and we all have a basic human need for recognition and involvement. We must have this need validated at very regular intervals. If you are not doing it with finance, you had better be doing it in other more demonstrative ways.

A Change for Change's Sake

I am suggesting throughout this chapter that you change things at regular, or even better, irregular intervals. I am suggesting you become truly eclectic in your approach to management; that you develop as many styles as you have employees. In this atmosphere of constant change and renewal it is most important that you test the cohesion of your staff system before, during and after each of the new developments (Anderson, 1997). It will by now be apparent, especially after this last statement, that I believe very strongly in the effects created by small changes which are regularly planned and implemented. Am I advocating that you make change for change's sake? Yes I am. Freshness and innovation are important team characteristics and also contribute to the emergence of a new culture.

Organisations that do the same things year after year become stale, stagnant and, worst of all, out of touch. Their players become afraid of new adventures. Fortress defence mentality allows the bonding needs of the regular group to set the template for the future. Newcomers are often made to feel intrusive and new ideas are afforded the same treatment.

Changes however, whether new influxes of staff, systematic manoeuvres, new models, new approaches, timetables or working practices, all help to keep the team fresh and on their toes. But change must also encompass the manager. Everything else cannot be changed around, and the manager remain the same. They must also be flexible and this may mean trying new management models or approaches and being open to constant feedback.

One of the ways I accomplish this is to write to each staff member individually at six-month intervals (or less if large change is planned) and ask them for their honest opinions. I ask this in writing and provide a format for them to reply. One of the questions I use to facilitate some guided replies is 'How am I doing?'. I often also include a gradient line for staff to show me graphically where they think we are in our quest for excellence.

I	2	3	4	5	6	7	8	9	10

On the line above please indicate to me, using your 'gut feeling',
where we are in achieving our goal of activity provision?

Some of the questions I ask are open like the one above and rely on 'gut' feelings. Others are more pointed and ask questions like: Did we achieve 65 per cent attendance at last month's training sessions? Each is designed to allow all of us a temperature check on how we are doing as a team. These questionnaires are important, as they allow a different perspective to surface than that shown in the open weekly meetings where people pursue their own acting job and play their own version of politics. None of us is the same 'true self' in a group situation, particularly a work group situation, as that 'self' we portray in the security and safety of our own homes. Even the most open and honest of people slips into a role when the metaphorical lights, camera and action begin.

A Possible Future Model may already be in Genesis

One model of care that allows us a possible glimpse of what these future care homes may look like in their approach, and which blends a number of styles, ideologies and techniques, is the Gentlecare approach (Jones, 2000), prominent throughout North America and Canada. When first coming across this system, many practitioners feel an almost instant empathy with its commonsense and inclusive approach. It was created by a woman who nursed her father until he died, and then created a style of care she wished to see practised for all other elders in the future. It is a stylised system of care programmes that at the least offers positive hope and inspiration as a guideline. Gentlecare seems to offer a workable model that encompasses many of the traits we should be looking to provide in good care homes.

Gentlecare takes a 24-hour approach to each individual, and works by creating programmes that fill up each hour of the waking day (no room for learned helplessness here). If we accept that a number of abilities may be lost as people increasingly need care, then leaving them to occupy themselves or provide their own active stimulation should not be seen as an option. Using a life history and present preferences and abilities model, Gentlecare allows the formation of daily activity and occupational programmes. These programmes do not just start at 1000 and finish at 1600, but are 24-hour commitments to engagement. Gentlecare views occupation as being the essential factor in providing happiness and staving off the ravages of increasing confusion or despair. The staff know and are involved with every individual and time is given to meeting each need. The needs of the establishment as such are placed on hold, or at least prioritised lower than the care of the individual. Things change constantly in these regimes and the vision is very compelling.

Earlier I stated that all staff members, all team members, should be involved in the care regime. The approach that I am advocating (and indeed is advocated by Gentlecare) means kitchen staff working to the person's individual preferences, involving the person in planning and, where possible, creating the menus and the meals; where housekeepers work alongside the residents in the cleaning and tidying; where the maintenance man has help from within, and where care staff share the goals of daily living with the residents as partners and not as custodians.

In Closing

There are no secrets to good management, but there are principles. Good principle-centred management (Covey, 2000) is about moral thinking, a good work ethic and a belief in the power of a collection of motivated, well-trained and well-rewarded people.

Occupation means being deeply immersed and involved in the current activity. To provide staff who are deeply immersed in their work, they need to see the benefits to themselves, as well as to the residents they are involved with. A regime where the manager leads the team by inclusion is just such an approach that aims to provide immersion by actively seeking contributions, opinions, directions and guidance from everyone, at every level. This has to be the way of the future. I have tried to lead without adopting this approach, and have failed on more than one occasion.

This new culture care system can only come about when the manager takes the ultimate responsibility for leading us into the care homes of the future. To do this they need to know their staff, their residents and, most importantly, themselves. Without a deep commitment to the well-being of all involved, the manager loses before he or she starts.

To close what I hope has been a passionate and spirited call to arms, I will recap some of the main points that may have escaped headings. Older people have a past, a present and a future. No care regime should be a place to come and die – except for hospices. Good staff must receive emotional value to give emotional support. When the wage is not great, the system must support, nurture and cushion. Managers who neglect this truth risk losing the best of staff to more enlightened competition. Only the best care homes will survive in the future and only the best staff will work in them. Care settings are suffering through increased bureaucracy. Enlightened managers should cut through this and provide a personal service to all in their care. If the manager feels isolated and misunderstood, perhaps the fault lies inside and not outside. After all, everyone is searching for someone to take an interest. Managers should strive to be a real life resource, not just a figurehead. Great care needs great people and every great team needs a great leader – stand up and be counted.

I referred earlier to having people share your vision and come on board with your way of thinking. Make your vision their vision. Create desire, paint a picture of the future and the road to it, and then work tirelessly until everyone shares the same goals. Always involve, always consult and make every individual feel important. When you give, you receive – give nothing and expect nothing in return.

For all you leaders and visionary managers out there, I salute you. Many of you are already doing these things – if you are not, give it a go. What have you got to lose except perhaps your best staff and the hope of those you care for?

CHAPTER 5

Successful Activity Planning

Hazel May

OUR THERAPEUTIC USE OF ACTIVITIES for people in care settings stems from certain widely held cultural values relating to engagement and well-being. We need to be mindful of this when approaching the job of activity provision if we are to ensure that our interventions are effective. 'Off the shelf' activity programmes may or may not be effective; they do not automatically result in engagement and well-being for the people at whom they are targeted. Individual activity plans derived from individual assessments are far more likely to be effective, and group programmes should ideally be rationalisations of individual plans. In this chapter I will outline a value base for effective activity interventions, and then discuss the key principles for assessment and activity planning.

A Value Base for Activity Provision

It is increasingly understood in health and social care settings today that human well-being arises from being recognised and treated as a unique person (Kitwood, 1997), and from being actively engaged with the world around us (Bradburn, 1969; Glass et al, 1999; Perrin & May, 1999). In care settings where individuality is not appreciated or addressed and/or where prolonged states of disengagement are observed, there is no question that, at best, well-being is compromised and, at worst, a person's psychological and emotional survival is placed under threat. There is ample research evidence available that disengagement from an active lifestyle is at the root of much of the ill-being we so often see in people living in long-term care settings (Armstrong-Esther et al, 1994; Nolan et al, 1995; Perrin 1997).

For this reason, the value base for activity provision should be derived from the concept of human engagement. The rationale for using activities is to engage people with the world around them, so that their well-being is sustained, and their experience of being treated and recognised as a unique person is upheld. Effective activities should result in positive engagement with a person, task or object. If the activity is effective, the well-being of the person will improve. If the person is disengaged or they start to show signs of ill-being, then the whole point is being missed, the activity is not effective and should be reviewed. In the example below, the activity worker has not planned her activity, and she knows nothing about the people she is trying to work with.

Unplanned Activity

A nursing home manager decided to hire an entertainer for the afternoon. She had seen the entertainer perform before and had been impressed by her sunny personality and musical skill.

The entertainer duly arrived after lunch and was shown into a medium-sized lounge where she proceeded to set up her musical instruments (an accordion and a guitar) and her sheet music. Various residents were escorted into the lounge and helped into two rows of seats facing the entertainer. The first row had been placed approximately five feet away from the entertainer in a 'concert style' arrangement.

I was sitting in the lounge observing at the same time, and saw that only two of the twelve residents who had been seated by staff in the lounge were engaging with the entertainer. One lady was passively watching and listening, and one man was clapping in time with the music. Half of the remaining ten fell asleep; two were distressed and showing signs of wanting to leave; three were awake but disengaged, either staring into space or sitting in a slumped position.

In this scenario, the entertainer needed help from the manager, and probably other workers in the home, to understand the needs and limitations of the people she was trying to engage with. Sadly, this is not an uncommon situation and reflects the old culture thinking that 'any activity is better than none', which results in the consequent action of ploughing on regardless. It was evident to me at the time that the manager felt she had gone beyond the call of duty to have organised and funded the event; that the care workers were grateful for somebody else to be reducing the demands upon them and that the entertainer saw the session as 'a good job done'.

The Process of Assessment

Common reasons for ineffective activities such as the one described above are:

- that communication is misunderstood or not understood;
- that the activity does not find its way into the person's world or is pitched at the wrong level.

Undertaking an individual assessment will help the activity provider to devise the means to communicate in a way the person can understand, and to pitch the activity at a level the person can engage with. An activity worker may not have the same level of knowledge and expertise as a psychologist, doctor, nurse or professional therapist. Nevertheless, it should be perfectly possible for activity workers to make their own full and comprehensive assessment. Such an assessment will provide the basis for successful activity plans.

Sources of information

As an activity worker, you will need to draw from a number of sources to gather the information you require to design an activity plan for Mr Waites.

Assessment Plan for Mr Waites

1 **The person.** Spend time communicating with and observing Mr Waites. What actions does he engage in naturally and without help? How does he communicate? Do you notice small things that help him to engage with his world?

2 **Family and friends.** What do they think he would like to do? What can they tell you about what he has enjoyed before? What activities have his relatives or friends tried to do with Mr Waites?

3 **Other staff and professionals.** Are there assessments that have already been done? These might throw light on particular abilities and disabilities that are relevant to activity planning. For example, hearing, visual or mobility problems, or difficulties with speaking/ understanding.

From Assessment to Plan

In this section Mr Waites will be used as a case example. An explanation of each aspect of his assessment will be provided along with examples (shown in boxes) of summaries and activity plan notes. Planning successful individual activities demands that the activity worker take a really close look at each person's uniqueness:

1 Personality
2 Health

3 Biography
4 Cognitive Capacity

Personality

Personality has a strong influence on engagement. Some people are shy and others extrovert; some people are domineering and others are not; some people like being with a group, while others prefer their own company. Some people become quiet and still when they are frightened or unsure, while others become angry and aggressive. Personality traits do not necessarily disappear when a person becomes ill, frail or goes into care; they may become exaggerated or masked by certain symptoms. It is likely that some of the quieter personalities in the example of the music session found the experience of being placed in a large group too overwhelming, while the man with the extrovert, confident personality clapped and sang along.

PERSONALITY
Mr Waites has been a domineering, conscientious and hard-working individual. He likes both his own company and being in 'the right kind' of group. He has a slapstick sense of humour and tends to confront people and situations if he is unhappy.

Notes for Activity Plan
Mr W will need to feel in control and be offered choices wherever possible. He might become confrontational if unhappy.

Health

Some physical conditions cause excessive sleeping. Depression can also cause excessive sleeping, as well as poor concentration and motivation. There may be physical reasons preventing a person from engaging in activity such as pain, discomfort or disability. How many of the residents who were staring blankly into space in the musical activity were hard of hearing? How many were slumping because of a physical condition such as arthritis? How could these residents possibly see what was happening from a slumped position?

HEALTH

Mr Waites is a strongly built, tall man. He has arthritis in his right ankle and a heart condition. Getting out of his chair is effortful, and he becomes breathless on exertion. He also has poor hearing in his right ear.

Notes for Activity Plan

- Short sessions lasting perhaps not more than ten minutes.
- Individual and group sessions where people can talk to him from his left side.
- Easy-to-do sitting activities (eg, dominoes, darts, shoe or silver polishing).

Biography

The things that have happened in the past dramatically affect how we behave in the here and now. Even though some age-related conditions may cause a person to be less able to recall facts, feelings can still arise by association. For example, a certain song can evoke powerful positive or negative feelings without any accompanying rational thinking. The sight of something can induce feelings of panic or fear. I knew of a man living in a residential home who often became aggressive and uncooperative during dressing in the morning. It emerged, as a result of looking into his biography, that he was frightened of water. The flooring in his room was shiny blue lino and the sight of the floor, which to him looked like water, was causing his response. Perhaps one of the distressed ladies in the musical activity was experiencing feelings arising from past experiences which were triggered by the music.

BIOGRAPHY

Mr Waites was the oldest of five children born into a working-class Irish Catholic family. He lived in London during the war years as a child, left school at 14, and joined the RAF where he worked as a PE Instructor. He was posted to Scotland where he met his wife. They moved to the south of England where they raised a family of four children. Mrs Waites stayed at home and Mr Waites worked in an insurance office in the City of London. His hobbies included music, old films (westerns), golf and travelling. He moved to live in the USA when his marriage broke down. At age 50, he remarried and continued to work in insurance until he retired 15 years later. He remained in the USA until he needed long-term care and his wife could no longer cope. At this stage he moved back to the UK where arrangements were made for him to move into a residential home near to one of his daughters.

Notes for Activity Plan

Visual, auditory and discussion themes and items could include:

• Material from old westerns
• Scotland, London, USA material
• Golf items and materials
• Music from his era – Beatles/jazz
• Modes of travel
• Activities of value to him might include:
  – Physical exercise
  – Office tasks.

Cognitive Capacity

Each person's capacity for doing is different. We all have physical and cognitive 'givens' that dictate to a large extent what we can and cannot do. A fit and healthy man weighing 14 stone and measuring 6 feet tall will be able to carry and move heavy objects and to walk long distances, whereas an older man, suffering from heart disease and of a much smaller physical frame, will have less capacity for this type of activity (these aspects of the assessment are discussed in the above section on health). On the other hand, the older man may have a much greater cognitive capacity than the younger for engaging in and doing well at complex card games such as bridge. Our physical and cognitive capacities are unique. For people living in care settings, it is not unusual for physical or cognitive capacity to alter, and to continue to alter, as time progresses.

Cognitive capacity refers to the extent of our thinking ability, and our thinking controls many of the things that we do in day-to-day life. Some dementing conditions such as Alzheimer's disease and vascular dementia affect the cortex of the brain. This is the part that enables us to think, analyse and plan in a conscious sense (ie, to know that we are thinking, analysing or planning). The lower brain, however, is often not affected, and so the emotional and primitive responses of a person are still very much intact.

Think of a small child of 'toddling' age; the child's cortex is not yet fully developed. This means that he is not yet able to engage with his world in a strictly cognitive way (ie, primarily through his thinking). He is not planning or analysing. He does not think consciously about what he is doing. He simply 'does', living through his hands and body. Yet his engagement with the world around him is masterful and his well-being is high. He engages in activities such as rolling, climbing, digging and generally playing.

In working with people in care settings who have damage to their cerebral cortex, it should be possible to facilitate experiences that are as fulfilling and enjoyable as that of the child described above. To do this, a basic understanding of cognitive development, ie, of how our thinking ability develops, is helpful. Popular theories are based on the idea that our cognitive ability develops from birth to maturity in stages, and that each stage has to be reached by the individual before they are able to progress to the next stage. This is rather like the 'can't run before you can walk' idea. One model currently being used by some occupational therapists working with people who have cognitive disabilities adopts this idea of stages, and suggests six levels of ability (Allen, 1985). Using this model, it is possible to identify at which level of ability the person is functioning, so that suitable and achievable activities can be planned.

People who do not have cognitive problems should be able to function at Level 5 and/or Level 6. At Level 6, the highest level of functioning, a person is capable of learning and able to plan ahead, anticipating the consequences of his or her actions. At Level 5, the capacity for planning and anticipating consequences is less advanced, but the ability for new learning is well-developed. Commonly, these higher cognitive abilities are the first to be affected by dementing conditions in older people. The consequent changes in the person's handling of day-to-day activities are not noticed. If they are, they are often accepted as simply a part of getting older.

The most common levels identified among older people needing residential or nursing care are Levels 1 to 4. It is not unusual, in the author's experience, for the older person with cognitive disabilities gradually to move through the stages from Level 4 to Level 2 once admitted to a nursing or residential home. It is rare to find people whose functioning has deteriorated to Level 1. A person at this level would probably be bed-bound. Here is a description of the Levels 1 through 4, which essentially mirrors human cognitive development from birth.

Level 1: Automatic action
A person with cognitive disabilities assessed at this level will have similar abilities to a small baby, and the capacity to engage with their world

through 'automatic' actions such as sucking, making eye contact and responding to external stimuli like bells, voices, pictures and mobiles.

Level 2: Postural action

At this level, the person with cognitive disabilities engages with his world primarily through his body. This is called postural action. The person is able to sit up, stand up and walk, and to push and pull objects to help achieve mobility; all this, of course, in addition to the abilities described in Level 1.

Level 3: Manual action

At this level, in addition to being able to engage in automatic action and postural action, the person is very interested in objects and wants to discover the world through his hands; picking things up, moving them, tasting them, rolling them, dropping them. Single step, repetitive manual activities are achievable for the person at this level.

Level 4: Goal-directed action

Automatic actions, postural and manual actions are well within the person's ability at this level. Additionally, the person can undertake some simple activities of daily living independently, such as doing up shoelaces, eating with a knife and fork, getting dressed. This is called goal-directed action.

Looking back at Mr Waites' life in the years leading to his admission to the care home, his decline in cognitive ability becomes apparent:

Mr Waites' Cognitive Ability

When Mr Waites retired, he decided to use some of his savings to make an annual visit home to England to visit his family. Each year, Mr Waites returned home to England for a few weeks. He usually travelled in the autumn, but would start his planning in the spring. This involved shopping around for good deals on air fares, making telephone calls to each individual niece and nephew to plan an itinerary that suited them and didn't interfere with their work and family commitments, and then piecing everything together. He would then type out a plan for each family member and send it ahead of his arrival. His family in England first noticed a change when, for the first year ever, he failed to send a plan. He talked, ahead of time, in general terms about his visit and gave his arrival details before he left, but that was all. Only by chance, the day before he was due to arrive, did one of his daughters realise that nobody had been asked to collect Mr Waites from the airport. She quickly organised the situation and her brother collected him. The visit didn't go too well this time because Mr Waites hadn't arranged with each family member how long he would be staying. Last-minute plans had to be made and this caused confusion, inconvenience, and sadly two of Mr Waites' daughters fell out over a misunderstanding about the arrangements. Nobody realised it at the time, but this visit marked the onset of Mr Waites' dementia. He was losing his capacity for **planned action**.

Mr Waites' favourite hobby had always been music. He loved listening to all sorts of modern and classical music. His taste and his collection were wide ranging, including all of the Beatles music and much treasured old jazz music. He took it upon himself after retirement to make tapes for various family and friends in England. On the tapes he enjoyed mixing a little bit of talking with different tracks of music from his own collection. He usually managed to send off one tape to England each month. About six months after his return from holiday in England the tapes stopped.

The reason for this related to a retirement gift! On his retirement from the company, he was presented with a new 'midi system' which he had postponed using. He wasn't too sure about how to rig it up. By chance he mentioned this to a neighbour who offered the help of her son to install the new system and show Mr Waites how to operate it. Just before Christmas, the young man had finally found time to call on Mr Waites and switch the midi system for the old one. This he did very quickly before spending half an hour or so showing Mr Waites how to use it. Mr Waites struggled to get the hang of the new system straightaway, but the neighbour's son left the instruction book out for him and felt sure that, with a little practice, he would eventually be able to use the new machine.

The old hi-fi was boxed up and stored in the attic. Unfortunately Mr Waites wasn't able to learn how to use the new midi system, despite several attempts. He kept making the same mistakes over and over again. He managed sometimes to play music, but not to tape it, because when he pressed the button that the neighbour's son had shown him, it flashed up 'play'. Mr Waites couldn't solve the problem, and was unable to learn that he needed to keep his finger on the button for longer to move the mode on to 'tape'. Mr Waites didn't worry too much. He felt he was losing interest anyway in making tapes, and that the children were probably old enough now to make their own if they wanted to. Mr Waites was losing his drive and ability for **exploratory action**. This, in turn, was affecting his ability to learn and to solve problems. Gradually, his range of activities and outings was diminishing.

Despite his struggle with planned action and exploratory action, Mr Waites was still living successfully at home. He was still able to do routine tasks inside and outside the home in familiar environments. However, slowly, problems emerged as he failed to keep track of less routine jobs, such as having his trousers and jackets dry-cleaned, paying bills, having his eyes tested, visiting the dentist, and keeping up his prescription for his heart tablets. His world was becoming smaller as he began to avoid new experiences, such as day trips with the church group. Gradually, Mr Waites was relinquishing certain roles both within his marriage (doing the 'man's' work) and in his community (chairman of the golf club). His contact with family back home was also being affected. By spring the following year, he decided not to go to England for his annual trip. When one of his nieces phoned, he told her that he would perhaps come next year but that he couldn't afford to visit annually any more.

Of course, changes of this nature in a person are very subtle. Many people and friends might not notice anything amiss, but the person experiencing a profound change in themselves may feel deeply anxious, knowing that something is wrong, but not understanding exactly what it is. As was the case with Mr Waites, many aspects of daily living remained unaffected, and he was still able to engage easily in certain types of occupation, such as day-to-day food shopping, making tea, making his bed and keeping his small garden in order.

On a very hot day that summer, while he was playing golf, Mr Waites had a heart attack and was rushed into hospital. During his recovery on the medical ward, staff noticed that he seemed disorientated and distressed. However, they put this down to the combined effects of the anaesthetic and the new drugs. In due course he was discharged home, only to be admitted again three weeks later in a state of self-neglect and with a broken wrist. He had fallen in the night, and had put his hand out to break the fall. This time the medical team referred Mr Waites to the local psychogeriatric team, and, within a week or so, a diagnosis of vascular dementia was confirmed. The team managed to support Mr Waites at home for a further 12 months, but finally it was apparent that he couldn't cope, and residential care was set up.

Now, two years later, having moved back to England and living in a residential home, Mr Waites spends his time walking around and touching things. He needs help to get dressed, but can manage each step with verbal prompting. He is gradually losing his ability and his drive to engage in **goal-directed action,** although he clearly enjoys handling objects and doing things with his hands. In terms of his ability to engage in occupation, he could be described as being in the **manual action** phase. He also hums old jazz tunes and Beatles songs as he fiddles and potters, and seems happily absorbed doing this.

PERSONALITY

Mr Waites needs help to complete goal-directed activities such as dressing, but he enjoys using his hands to pick up, explore and move objects.

Notes for Activity Plan

• Help Mr Waites to engage in routine daily activities, such as dressing, food preparation.

• He should still be able to hit a golfball (? check).

• Cleaning and handling of golf items.

• Sensory, creative activities with no rules or particular end result, such as pottery, painting.

• Singing and dancing.

Theories and models provide important and helpful frameworks for planning activities but, most importantly, you should spend time watching out for all the things that the person can do, and make notes so that you do not forget. These abilities may not be apparent during planned activities sessions or when the person is asked to do them. In other words, do not assume that a person who does not do certain things when asked cannot do those things at all.

Sample Activity Plan

Here is a sample activity plan for Mr Waites, that has used all the information gathered during the assessment process. Note that the activity plan includes strategies for improving Mr Waites' engagement with everyday activities such as dressing.

Activity Plan for Mr Waites

1 All activities should be offered to Mr Waites with at least one alternative choice.

2 Smaller select groups are likely to be more successful, eg, men's discussion group and physical exercise group.

3 Physical sessions should be short, lasting perhaps not more than ten to fifteen minutes.

4 During individual and group sessions, other people should talk to him from his left side.

5 Physical activities should be gentle, such as sitting and standing activities using ball or balloon. Physical fitness exercises may be familiar to him, but need to be adapted to suit his current ability.

6 Visual, auditory and discussion themes and items could include:
   • material from old westerns
   • Scotland, London, USA material
   • golf items and materials
   • music from his era – Beatles/jazz
   • modes of travel.

7 Activities of value to him might include:
   • physical exercise
   • office tasks
   • he should still be able to hit a golf ball (? check)
   • cleaning and handling of golf items.

8 Mr Waites should be helped and encouraged to engage in routine daily activities, such as dressing, self-care activities and food preparation; also sensory and creative activities with no rules or particular end result, such as pottery, painting, singing and dancing.

Reviewing your Plan

Activity plans need to be reviewed for two reasons: first, to check that they have been effective; second, to ensure that they are updated should the person's health or cognitive capacity change. As discussed at the start of this chapter, effectiveness relates to engagement and well-being, so your review will need to include some measure of these. This can be done informally, through observation and discussion with the person, staff and family, or more formally, using a structured method such as Dementia Care Mapping (Innes & Surr, 2001) or the Bradford Dementia Group's Well/Illbeing Profile (Bruce, 2000). As part of the work, activity workers need to agree arrangements for regular review with the rest of the team. This will require discussion and agreement about how often reviews should be undertaken, and who should be involved.

Returning to the scenario where the entertainer attempted to engage with the group, it is clear that the activity was inadequately resourced. A more successful activity would have been part of a much larger process. There was a lack of planning, and so the activity lacked any 'value base'. The manager and care home staff, those with in-depth knowledge about the people in the group, left the entertainer to get on with it. Not surprisingly, the session did not provide an opportunity for the individuals in the group to experience being recognised and treated as special, unique people. The session failed to bring about engagement. It did not improve well-being for most of the individuals, and could therefore be judged, at best, to be a waste of resources, and, at worst, to have been damaging for some people. In missing a crucial part of activity provision – assessment and planning – the home was (inadvertently perhaps) engaging in old culture values and practices, and endorsing the 'slumped-in-the-lounge' lifestyle for the people living there.

A session that had been planned, taking into account each person's uniqueness, would have been different. A session that included reflecting on each person as part of its process, noticing signs of distress and disengagement, and finding out more about each individual, would have been more successful. A successful session would have been adequately resourced, allowing time for the staff involved to make individual assessments and continuously to review, reflect and adapt their approaches. These staff would then be in a good position to help others (like the entertainer) to adapt their approach; for example, by suggesting that the entertainer use her time to offer three very short sessions with individuals, or to work 'close range' with a much smaller group, encouraging and helping those involved to express themselves through singing, clapping or playing an instrument.

Successful activities are achievable in long-term care settings regardless of disability. As a result of devoting time to the process of assessment and planning for each individual, the value of all the activities in care settings, including day-to-day eating, dressing and self-care, can be greatly enhanced for all concerned. Life for people in care settings can, and should, be purposeful and enjoyable. The new culture of therapeutic activity is the means to this end.

CHAPTER 6

The Critical Importance of Biographical Knowledge

Charlie Murphy

THIS CHAPTER EXAMINES THE ROLE that knowledge of the individual's life story plays in therapeutic activity with older people, across all settings, but particularly with those who have memory problems. Life story work is an important activity, not just for the older person, but also for staff/volunteers who work with them and for family carers. This chapter outlines the benefits for all three groups, and offers some brief guidance on how one might go about starting life story work with someone. The chapter also includes a working definition of life story work.

In my post as development worker at the Dementia Services Development Centre, I am often asked to deliver activities training to front-line staff, usually in day-care or home-support situations. Staff and volunteers at these events often expect a shopping list of new activity ideas. Instead they get taken back to basics – why, who and what? So, rather than being given a list of new activities, they are asked to explore the reasons they carry out activities in the first place, and who they carry out activities with. I sometimes make the analogy of planning a meal for unexpected visitors. You would want to know the purpose that the meal was to serve (ie, the *why*); then *who* these visitors were, before rushing to the recipes. Similarly there is the need to know the person/people with whom you do activities.

Defining Life Story Work

> Life story work is about finding out, recording and making use of relevant facts from the individual life story – past and present – of the person.

I distinguish three interlinked 'tasks' in doing life story work:

- finding out;
- recording;
- making use of the life story work.

It is important to stress that the 'finding out' need not be an additional, separate, highly demanding piece of work. Often workers already know some biographical information to start with. This may have been recorded on a referral form; perhaps a family carer, during a discussion on a family background, may have provided it; or it could have come directly from the individual concerned, perhaps in a quiet moment of shared activity or a reminiscence session. The recording of the life story is important to ensure the information is available to more than one person – and available for the individual themselves in the case of dementia. One worker I spoke to felt that he carried around life story *images* of the people that he worked with. Life story work encourages workers to make such images more concrete. Finally, there is the need to make use of the life story work. It will not be of much benefit to gather the information and then leave it in a folder, unused.

Another important aspect of the above definition is that life story work concerns itself with information on 'personally relevant' parts of the life story. There does not need to be a checklist of headings that might constrain us all within neat boxes. In adopting such an approach parts of the 'story' are devoted to childhood, to family, to work, to hobbies, to holidays and to travel, for example. However, recognising that we are all individuals demands that we approach the life story in a unique way. Things that might be important for the worker, such as hobbies and family, might not be as important to the service user.

Notice also that we talk about the past and the present – that is 'story' as opposed to 'history'. This is partly an acknowledgement that the person's story continues. It is not over because the person has retired or has dementia. Also the story should have a future: what are the person's wishes for the future, secret daydreams or ambitions?

Benefits of Life Story Work for Service Users

This section outlines the major benefits for the person themselves if workers take the time to do some life story work with them. These benefits apply to all older people, and especially to individuals with dementia.

Reinforcing sense of identity/self

Our memories, our story, provide so much of our identity and our sense of self. In many long-stay care homes, we see elderly women attaching great importance to their handbags. For men it might be a familiar walking stick. Consider the experience of long-stay care from their point of view. These objects are some of the very few things which are personal, which give them a sense of identity. They sit in a room much larger than any they have been used to, in a building larger than any they have lived in before, with many strangers and unfamiliar routines to adjust to. Is it so surprising that a familiar handbag, hat or walking stick can acquire such significance?

A worker who attended one of my training courses talked of an individual she had worked with in day care. Together they had produced a life story book for this person. Subsequently he had moved to long-stay care. Although his dementia had deteriorated to the extent that he could not use much of the book independently, he fastidiously carried it with him, tucked under his arm, when he walked around the home. He knew that the life story book conveyed an important sense of self and identity. The following extract from a conversation which the writer John Killick had with an individual with dementia illustrates this pointedly: 'I often wonder why people bother with people like us. I could have reeled it off for what you are doing. It's a life story. It's the biography of the person you are writing about. It's me'. In this instance, the speaker sees no distinction between talking about his story and his actual identity. The American researcher, Habib Chaudhary, also elaborated on this issue when he stated, 'Self-identity and personal meaning get largely overtaken by institutional policies and routines' (2002, p42).

Improving self-esteem
Life story work can function in a number of ways to improve self-esteem. First, there is the boost we can receive from others who show interest in aspects of our life. Reminiscence professionals often talk about passing on traditions, where the older person acts as a conduit for keeping the experiences of their generation alive. At the same time, workers are validating the individual's past experiences.

Second, there is the opportunity for the person to share their experiences and to give something back. Older people, and people with dementia in particular, can often feel that they are solely recipients in the care environment, having no chance to reciprocate, whether to staff or to other users. A story told by them to an interested group about their own life experience can be an important opportunity to 'give'. I know of one day centre where life story work with a male attendee uncovered a very keen interest in pigeon fancying. This man, normally quite reticent, talked extensively about his hobby. As a result, his 'talk' on pigeon fancying was occasionally scheduled as an activity at the centre. So this man had regular opportunities to share his enthusiasm and knowledge about his subject with a group of interested people – the opportunity to contribute, to give back.

Coleman et al (1993) also speak of the importance of self-esteem in helping someone to tackle major life-changing events that could pose a threat to their sense of identity.

Failure-free activity

Ultimately we are all the experts on our own lives. Hence talking with someone about their life story, and compiling or using a piece of life story work with the person, are activities that the person cannot fail at. This can be particularly important for individuals with dementia, who can be confronted with so many failures in their lives as their dementia progresses. The advantage of life story work is that, with the right kind of interaction, the person is able to regain a sense of achievement and recognition. One warning here is that the life story work should not be used as a test for someone who has memory problems. If so, it moves away from being a failure-free activity.

Enjoyment

Life story work has the potential to be an enjoyable activity. During the experiential exercise that I run as part of life story work training courses, participants' voices are always very animated as people who are often strangers to one another engage in short discussions about their own life story, based on a photograph which they have brought along.

This is not to argue in favour of ignoring sad events in the person's past. Often the prospect of uncovering unhappy memories can present the greatest difficulties for workers in this field. There can be a tendency for workers to change the subject, to hide away from such experiences. Yet we all have faced sadness in our lives. For older people there may have been less opportunity at the time to express such emotions and to talk about sad events. When such memories are recalled through life story work, it may be the first time that this person has shared the memory with another. Perhaps all that they require is to be listened to. Some workers may feel that they have to 'fix' the problem and thus feel daunted. However, the older person may simply be asking for a sympathetic hearing. One worker who attended a training course talked of a resident in the home where she worked who would often pace around agitatedly, saying 'I wasn't there, I wasn't there'. This worker, who was quite new, decided to try to explore the resident's story. They had tea in a quiet room and talked about the person's background. It was here that the woman revealed that her mother had died when she was still a child of nine or ten. It was not the accepted custom for children to attend funerals at that time, so she was prevented from doing so. This event had distressed her greatly and stayed with her. Talking with the worker, the resident was able to fully express her feelings around this event. Together they shared tears over the loss. One outcome was that the resident was no longer distressed about not 'being there'.

Reinforcing long-term memory
The multi-sensory prompts that workers can use in life story folders to help recollect past events may be very valuable. These prompts, such as photographs, tactile objects, musical or other sounds, encourage the retention and recall of longer-term memories. This has especial relevance for individuals with dementia. A nursing home manager in Glasgow recalled how one resident who had been widowed for a long time and did not mention her late husband's name reacted to his de-mob photograph in her life story book with great pleasure, and recalled details seemingly long forgotten.

Maintaining/building up relationships with paid/unpaid carers

Relationships between staff and residents in care settings can often revolve around the care practice and the routines of the setting. People talk about when lunch will come and what will be on the menu. Even in the community such interactions can take on a vague 'one size fits all' quality. Workers talk in generalities, having little personal background to base other conversation around. Life story work allows relationships to become more personal, more individually focused. This should, of course, be a two-way process. Workers have the opportunity to share something of their life story and their background in return. For some professionals this can go against their notions of professional distance. Yet is it not presumptuous to expect the older person to disclose aspects of themselves without some reciprocity (Kitwood, 1997)? Also, for individuals with dementia, staff might assume that a particular conversation/statement is meaningless if they do not have the life story/biographical context to set it in or relate it to. Thus opportunities for a more involved interaction can be lost.

This benefit applies also to relationships with unpaid carers, family and friends. A worker at a training course in Nottingham spoke of receiving a call from a close friend of one of her clients, whom the worker had recently helped with her move into long-stay care. The friend, who lived in the north of England, was coming to visit this woman in the home for the first time. She was anxious about what they would talk about. The worker suggested the visitor bring along some photographs from their joint past (they had both performed on the stage). The outcome was that both friends enjoyed a very pleasant couple of hours in each other's company. Their relationship was able to re-establish itself from this beginning.

Reinforcing social skills

Social skills can diminish if they are not being put to use. Situations where older people can feel comfortable and confident in conversation, such as their own life story, can help to preserve these abilities. Gemma Jones (quoted in Goldsmith, 1996, p56) talks of the 'nothing' conversations and vacuous pleasantries with which staff can engage residents in long-stay care situations. Consequently residents' capacity for conversation diminishes.

For older people with dementia, opportunities for conversation can be fewer simply because people (eg, old friends and extended family) no longer visit. These ex-visitors might be concerned that the person did not remember their previous visit, or that their visit is having no effect. They may be worried about what they can talk about, as discussion of current issues tails off due to the poor memory of the individual with dementia. One woman who cared for her mother tackled this by adapting a photograph album into a kind of life story book. She added some captions and annotations to the photographs, then had the album open at relevant pages: for example photographs which showed her mother and the visitor together. This had a dual purpose. The visitor had a point from which to initiate conversation and her mother had a cue to remind her who the visitor was.

Benefits of Life Story Work for Family Carers

This section outlines significant benefits for the family carers of older people if some life story work is started with their relative. These benefits apply for carers of all older people, but particularly carers of individuals with dementia.

Reinforces 'the whole person' for family carers, extended family

One carer I knew had been asked if she would be interested in producing, or helping to produce, a life story book for her mother who had just entered long-stay care. The home had a policy of encouraging life story work. The woman reflected on the request and decided very quickly that she would pass it on to her own teenage daughter. She felt that her daughter's view of her grandmother had been skewed by the older woman's more recent experiences. The teenage granddaughter knew her grandmother as this frail woman who had been in and out of hospital, had required substantial support to live at home, and who now had been admitted to a nursing home. The task of helping to compile her grandmother's life story gave the young girl greater insight into the totality of her grandmother's experiences and a fuller appreciation of her life. This possibility that life story work may re-establish the wholeness of someone's life is a very important benefit. It moves people on from being defined and constrained by their illness and/or their age.

Challenges the increased separation of carer and cared for
When one half of a couple develops an illness, especially something like dementia, it is possible that the relationship of carer and cared for becomes the predominant one in the partnership, superseding that of husband and wife, for example. Reclaiming or rediscovering the cared for person through their life story challenges this separation. A worker at a training course in Scotland who was also a daughter of someone with dementia talked of trying to encourage her father to produce a piece of life story work on his wife, ie her mother. However, her father was quite reluctant. He was very tired from caring for his wife. Recently she had been admitted to long-stay care so he was also having to deal with these emotions. Their sixtieth wedding anniversary was imminent and he had very little enthusiasm for it. One morning, however, he agreed to his daughter's suggestion that they take down the biscuit tin of old photographs and have a look through them. This happened at 10am. It was 12 hours before they put the tin away. Her father described the experience as 'the most enjoyable day he had spent in a long time'. What happened? The photographs had stirred memories of shared events with his wife: of their courtship, of achievements they had shared together, and of a sense of pride in raising their family. Furthermore the father now felt that he would like to do something to help his wife to record her life story, and indeed, to acknowledge and celebrate their forthcoming wedding anniversary.

Gives family carer a feeling of continued involvement

When an older person moves into long-stay care, the family carer may want to continue to be involved in that person's care, but feel that there are few opportunities for them to contribute. In some instances they may feel that their further contribution is unwelcome. A request from a worker, or indeed from their relative, to help in the development of a piece of life story work about the person, can restore that sense of involvement. The family carer can feel that they are playing an ongoing part in their relative's care in a very practical fashion. In his research Chaudhary quotes one worker who addressed this topic:

> This (biographical work) is a great way to involve families. Many family members want to be more involved and we don't always have things to do together … [it] can be an interesting way to involve the families. In fact, this way we can know the families better. (2002, p44)

Family carers' feelings of exclusion can also apply to day-care situations. Equally then, being asked to assist with the compilation of some life story work can have a role to play here.

Offers an activity to do at home

Some family carers can feel that their role revolves exclusively around practical and physical care tasks. This can be particularly true in caring for someone with dementia, for example. One carer on a training course talked of how she had her eyes opened to activities that she could share with her husband, who had dementia, at home. As he sat watching the Remembrance Day parades on television she relinquished the opportunity to get on with some housework and joined him. She recalled how he shared stories from his war days that she had never heard before.

Benefits of Life Story Work for Staff and Volunteers

This section outlines significant benefits for those working with older people in initiating life story work with the individual. These benefits apply to all older people, with the final one applying particularly to working with individuals with dementia.

Permits the planning and delivery of individual care

Best (1998) argues that the use of a biographical approach is 'imperative' in assessing the needs of an older person. Ultimately, the greater the knowledge and understanding that we have of the individuals that we work with, the more we will be able to deliver care and services that are tailored to that individual, rather than being tailored broadly to older people in general. One manager who attended a life story work training course felt that: 'it [life story work] gives you a better understanding of clients' individual needs ... we can write better individualised care plans'.

Similarly, a day hospital worker talked about the effect of doing life story work on the activities programme, commenting that it 'helped other staff to know the patients better and to plan further activities'.

Both remarks reinforce the point made by Chaudhary that 'biographical knowledge [promotes delivery of]... activities that are more meaningful than generic activities for all residents' (Chaudhary, 2002, p44). This is because workers can exploit their knowledge of clients' interests, background, past employment, hobbies and so on, in order to develop individually tailored activities.

In 1999 I carried out an evaluation of life story work at two nursing homes in Glasgow. Staff who were interviewed in this evaluation talked about four aspects of the impact which life story work had had on them:

1 Increased knowledge of the person;
2 Improved understanding of the person;

3 Changed attitudes towards the person;
4 Altered practice with the person.

All of the above can be seen as contributing towards the planning and delivery of individual care. Those who talked of increased knowledge were primarily hands-on staff. As one worker put it, residents' medical histories were meaningless to them, and without the life story material they did not know their residents 'from Adam'.

The second point, about improved understanding, was emphasised by both qualified and unqualified staff. One nurse commented: 'You can forget that they did have lives ... [the life story book] makes you take a step back ... they are not just old people waiting to be cared for.'

The classification of people as being limited or defined by their age and/or their disability surfaced frequently under this heading. It was as if having access to the life story expanded people beyond these limiting constraints in the eyes of those who worked with them. This was further elaborated by those workers who talked about how their attitudes had changed through having life story books in the homes. At its simplest the life story book enabled the staff to see 'people instead of patients'. One care worker put this in the context of the institutionalisation which can further corrode identity:

> You only see them as they are in these sort of places, but if you read through it [the book] you realise ... you forget they have been young before, been through the war – good times and bad times – especially if there are photos involved – you look at them in a different way.

In terms of changed practice one nurse summarised this by saying that she was a better nurse through having access to the life story of the people that she cared for.

Another study (Ross, 1990) involved a group of 25 professionals carrying out life review with older people. The group included both nurses and social workers. Participants observed that neither their professional training nor their clinical experience had given them the understanding and regard for their ageing patients which the process of gathering biographical information through life review had achieved. Additionally, they had a greater appreciation of the contribution that older people made to society.

Provides valuable information to other services such as long-stay care

Life story work can benefit staff across the services through which older people might move such as home support, day care, respite, long-stay care. In particular, the life story work or biographical information can help the person communicate aspects of their life story that they may have difficulty remembering in the progression through services. As mentioned in the previous section, such information may result in workers altering their attitudes towards the people with whom they work. Research by Pietrukowicz and Johnson (1991) illustrated how even a small amount of biographical information could alter the perspective and attitudes of professional nurses towards new admissions. Two groups of nurses were given the same information about a potential new admission, eg physical and medical details. However, the second group had an additional paragraph detailing some of the personal history of the referral. This second group showed more positive attitudes towards referrals/patients as a result of such additional insights.

Can build on previous coping strategies

In the Ross study (1990), previously referred to, the participants felt that they had gained an increased understanding of coping strategies used in the past by the older people with whom they worked. Significantly for the workers' own practice, this aspect of biographical knowledge could be put to use with their clients in helping them through illnesses or challenges which they currently faced. The importance, for both present and future practice, of hearing how people have coped in the past, has also been highlighted by Malcolm Johnson (1994).

Increased job satisfaction

We have already seen how life story work can enable staff to get to know the people that they work with better, and to look beyond disabilities and/or ageist attitudes. This is bound to help workers in their work, increasing the personal and individual nature of interactions, and giving value to the people with whom staff work. This point was also emphasised by Pietrukowicz and Johnson in the paper referred to above (1991).

Helps communication

The outcome or product of doing life story work is itself an aid to communicating with clients, members and users. Furthermore, familiarity with the contents of a given individual's life story work assists workers in their communication. One participant from a training course summarised this as 'more effective communication between service users and day centre staff'.

On a very practical level, a care worker who took part in the evaluation of life story work that I carried out in 1999 expressed similar sentiments when asked what she thought were the benefits of doing life story work in the nursing home where she worked. She felt that life story work promoted individually relevant communication:

You just get back a blank expression if you are not talking about something that they [the resident] recognise, so if you can go back to something from their past you get a wee something and it's nice to get that back.

An activity in itself

The process of collecting information in order to put together some life story work can provide an activity of its own for staff and service users. This would be especially important in ensuring that the completed item was a reflection of the person's own story and not someone else's telling of it. For example, some workers have talked of how family carers have helped to produce life story work that is their story of the life of the person they care for. Subsequently workers have had to work with the user to recraft the story.

Offers explanations from the past for present-day behaviours

For people with dementia some present-day behaviours may be better understood in the context of the person's past. A name called out plaintively at night-time may be that of a former beloved pet. Rising early in the morning may reflect that practice for 60 years as a farm labourer. Similarly, other seemingly meaningless behaviours may have their roots in the person's lifestyle or previous employment.

Other benefits

The research which I carried out on life story work produced the following additional responses from staff when asked why they used life story work:

- to have a non-institutional conversation;
- to improve mood if lonely, low, etc;
- for reality orientation purposes;
- to provide something that both can relate to;
- to offer something enjoyable from the person's past;
- for stimulation;
- for relaxation;
- to keep reminding the person;
- to explore likes and dislikes;
- to have something familiar to talk about.

How to Do Life Story Work

Space restrictions prevent a full exploration of how one might proceed with life story work – the assimilation of biographical information. A useful starting point would be for the worker to ask themselves why they are doing the life story work with the person in question. There could be a range of reasons taken from the various benefits already outlined. Clarity of purpose at the outset will enable the worker to monitor whether they have achieved what they set out to do.

Another important criterion in the compilation of life story work is to remain conscious of whose life story it is. This starts with obtaining the person's permission to proceed, and continues with their ongoing involvement and approval as the compilation of the story develops. As far as possible it should remain the person's own story.

For many people appropriate multi-sensory prompts are valuable in helping them to talk about their lives. Subsequently some of these prompts might be used in illustrating a part of the life story work. An emphasis on the communication of people's experiences and their meaning for them should remain paramount over the pursuit of possibly spurious pinpoint factual accuracy in the compilation of the story.

Summary

This chapter has attempted to remind readers of the key role that life story work can play in working with older people. I have illustrated and expanded on the numerous benefits which can flow from such work, whether to staff, family carers or the older person themselves. I will conclude with a response from a worker when asked what he thought were the reasons for doing life story work: 'to provide information for staff, and even relatives and the person themselves ... to show they are real people. They've had a life, some have had crackin' lives – good and bad times'.

CHAPTER 7

The Activity Coordinator: On the Way In or on the Way Out?

Vivienne Ratcliffe

What Does Activity Mean?

One dictionary definition of 'activity' is 'the state of being active; the exertion of energy'. For most of us this definition covers life in the workplace, general chores and the interests and hobbies that we enjoy in our spare time. We use energy mentally or physically in our work and play. However, perhaps we need to think in more detail about what we mean by activity in relation to people living in care environments. Those who have severe physical disabilities or suffer from dementia can still benefit from and enjoy activity, but 'the state of being active; the exertion of energy' is very often not possible. To promote activity in such an instance, we who care for them need to be active and to exert energy ourselves, in order to encourage their engagement with others or with the environment. Perhaps a better definition for our purposes is that activity in the care setting may be understood as engaging with the people, things and circumstances of our environment. Engagement can be positive and constructive, or negative, and it is important to clarify the difference. Positive engagement brings pleasure and contentment; negative engagement brings hostility, distress or apathy.

I once encouraged two gentlemen to share a game of dominoes, something they often enjoyed. They were friends and spent time together. While both started the game willingly, within a short time I could see that although one gentleman was full of enthusiasm, the other was clearly not happy. He did not become angry since he did not want to upset his friend, but he had really just wanted to doze. I had thought that he should be doing something. I was so wrong. I had engaged him negatively.

Activity should bring pleasure, stimulation, comfort, a sense of achievement and a sense of well-being. It is about being able to make decisions and have choice in how to spend each day. Activity should be encouraged, but not forced. It is unique to each individual, and is about friendship and laughter, about confidence and self-esteem. In our own lives we all come from different backgrounds, have different interests and enjoy the company of different people. Sometimes we do not really feel like doing much. We want to switch off from the world. To promote activity when those in our care feel like this is often to attempt to engage them negatively.

Constructive activity should always be a positive experience. Once while I was working in a home for people with dementia, a lady asked during a short communion service if she could read a psalm. She knew what she wanted to read and proudly stood, psalm book in hand, as we all sat and listened. Her sense of achievement at being involved in the service was a very positive experience – not only for her, but also for the staff involved and for the priest who was conducting the service. From that day onwards, communion services became much more about engagement with people, and not just simply about delivering spiritual care.

What Does the Title 'Activity Coordinator' Mean?

Most people have broadly the same understanding of the role of a nurse, a domestic assistant, or a chef. If I were to ask a cross-section of the public for definitions, I would expect that the replies would be very similar. I might be told that a nurse looks after people who are ill, she gives drugs, or that she is trained to care for the sick. A chef is someone who earns his living from cooking. A domestic assistant is someone who does domestic work, including cleaning. There are, however, many different perceptions and expectations of what an activity coordinator actually does.

At present, anyone can be employed as an activity coordinator. No training is required and no qualifications are mandatory. I believe that this is unacceptable and must change. The title of 'activity coordinator' should only be used by those who have undergone a specific period of training with a recognised body and who have gained a recognised national qualification. There must be standards for the role. The respect of other care professionals is essential if the activity coordinator is to be able to lead and coordinate activities within a home. The activity coordinator needs to be the leader in a specialist field, the person with the expertise to coordinate an overall plan of activity provision in a home.

I remember walking into a dining room at breakfast time in a home for people with dementia. One lady was sitting back in her chair with her arms folded, resolutely refusing to eat her breakfast. She was asking for 'brown stuff'. I knew that this lady had enjoyed a wonderful and varied social life and liked a sherry before lunch. The fact that it was breakfast time and not lunchtime was irrelevant to her. She was having a meal and wanted her customary sherry. I was fortunate to have a home manager whom I knew would support me in producing the sherry bottle at breakfast time. I poured a small glass and was rewarded with a huge smile and a 'Thank you, darling'. Breakfast, or at least part of it, was then eaten. Time was not wasted encouraging and cajoling, or, worse still, attempting to spoon-feed the lady. Leading and coordinating activities means being involved at other times of the day as well as conventional 'activity times', and using one's knowledge to ensure that residents are eating and enjoying their food and retaining their dignity.

To coordinate an overall plan of activity provision in a home means that the activity coordinator should be with different staff at different times throughout the day, leading, sharing knowledge, listening and observing. Ideally everyone participates, but the activity coordinator takes the helm, and tries to ensure that all residents are involved in activity provision in some way. The activity provision may be as simple as giving someone the opportunity to have sherry for breakfast.

It is fundamental to good practice in activities to remember that each of us is an individual and our needs and expectations are varied and diverse. For those living in a care environment there are basic rights that all are entitled to expect: the right to respect, dignity, privacy, kindness and comfort. The activity coordinator, in common with all other staff, must have these basic rights constantly in mind. The role requires a person who can, if necessary, make decisions on another's behalf, who can interpret need, gain trust, and be a friend to resident and relative alike.

I have often been told that 'My husband (or wife, father, mother) will not be able to take part in activities'. A common perception among relatives is that activities are about painting, woodwork, flower arranging and similar craft-based hobbies. The activity coordinator needs to explain that a culture of therapeutic activity embraces a far wider range of 'doing things' and, as a result, is able to change perceptions, encourage expectations, inspire confidence, and instil hope. To use a previous example; enjoying a sherry is an activity, and should be perceived as such – as a perfectly legitimate part of the lady's activity programme. The activity coordinator's role is one which should help reassure relatives that their loved ones, regardless of illness or disability, will be helped to lead a life which is about positive engagement with the people and environment in which they live.

In a care environment, how do the other staff perceive the activity coordinator's role? Unfortunately, this role is sometimes seen as being different from care, and yet in many ways they are one and the same thing. Caring for someone is about looking after the whole person. All who work in the care sector have something positive to offer in the way of activity.

Planned Activities

Planned group activities play an important role in any care home. Hopefully, a visitor walking in and seeing a hive of activity feels welcome and warmth. Craft sessions, baking, wine-making, gardening, poetry readings, and all the other many and varied group activities, need setting up and planning. Group sessions promote friendship and interaction, and enable people to enjoy a variety of different experiences. It is difficult at the present time to see how a care home without an activity coordinator could offer planned activities on a regular basis, given the pressure and constraints of the work of other staff. This does not mean that staff from other disciplines should not bring their ideas and/or contributions for planned activities to the activity coordinator. It is important that all staff are encouraged to be part of a forum for new ideas. If a member of staff has a particular skill or interest and wants to plan and run a group, then this should be welcomed.

Spontaneous Activities

Some of the best activity work often goes unnoticed. Seizing the moment for spontaneous activities offers opportunities for all disciplines in a care environment to contribute. Some people have innate skills which enable them to step in almost instinctively and to offer something really positive. In a busy care environment, staff have work that has to be finished and, sometimes because of the pressures, are able only to concentrate on the task in hand. Unfortunately, this means that opportunities for spontaneous activities can be lost. Such activities often last just a few minutes, but these minutes can dramatically change the way a person feels. Seeing someone tapping a foot to music enables any member of staff to interact and join in. Clapping, dancing, holding hands together – it does not matter what is happening – it is the interaction and the sharing that matters. Kneeling beside someone, stroking a face, smiling, making someone feel special – all take just a few moments. For most of us touch is a basic need. Those in care environments have the same needs as the rest of us. Sometimes perhaps, we fail to recognise ourselves in those we care for. The requirements that residents have for their physical care may blur our vision. If I am ever locked in my own world, rocking to and fro, possibly dribbling or incontinent, I do hope that someone will give me a hug, smile at me, and turn my chair to face the sun. I do hope that someone will have the time to pause and notice me, and will know that when I was well I did enjoy a gin and tonic.

Spontaneous activities sometimes require a lack of inhibition, demanding that one make a bit of a fool of oneself. I once walked into a sitting room in a dementia care environment intending to look for a book. It was a dull, dreary day, and the residents' spirits seemed low. I turned back and returned with a skipping rope. I started to skip. Within moments I was being watched, smiles began to appear, and the atmosphere in the room changed. One of the care staff watching my rather pathetic efforts, took the rope from me. He really *could* skip, and I stood back admiring his efforts. People were relaxing, laughing, showing pleasure and there was conversation. The sense of well-being was almost tangible. The whole experience only lasted about ten minutes, but was tremendously positive.

The old culture of activities was almost entirely group-orientated, and the new has become increasingly individualised. The value of group work should not be underestimated, but the new culture, with its emphasis on individual needs, means that there are expectations of activity provision for all. Spontaneous activities often reveal much of the best in the new culture.

Making the Most of Activities of Daily Living

Helping someone get up and get washed and dressed in the morning is usually the role of the care staff. Seeing this as an opportunity for interaction and activity, and not simply a task to be completed, is fundamental to a culture of therapeutic activity. Assisting someone to prepare for the day gives care staff an opportunity for engagement with residents on a totally individual basis. They enter into the private world of someone else – another person's bedroom, with that person's possessions, clothes and familiar objects. It is important that staff understand and respect the fact that, regardless of illness or disability, they walk into another human being's personal space. Talking, watching, listening and using every opportunity to try and promote activity, is a challenge for all who care. We choose the clothes that we wear each day ourselves, and it is essential that, if possible, the same choice is given to all those in care environments. For those who cannot articulate or choose for themselves, the responsibility of suitable choice is left to us. Talking about the clothes that have been chosen, or paying a compliment, engages the resident positively. Having a cup of tea together and sharing time helps relax and reassure. We all need to feel that, within the busy hub of life, people have time for us. The radio can be switched on with news or music appropriate to the individual. There can be little more soul-destroying than having someone tune your radio to a programme that you cannot stand, particularly first thing in the morning. Care staff have many opportunities for engagement and interaction as they enable those they help care for to start each new day. The uniqueness of each person's individual path through life provides a wonderful basis for activity.

There are the other activities/tasks that we all have to deal with as part of our daily life. We clean our homes, prepare food, lay tables, wash up, make beds, iron, cook – the list is endless. We write letters, pay bills, and do all sorts of different jobs in the house and garden. It is important that residents are given the chance to continue to perform these tasks of everyday life if they so choose. This is where it is possible for every discipline in every care situation to contribute to a culture of therapeutic activity. To look at how this can be put into practice we need to pick out areas of work performed by other staff.

The gardener

Residents can help choose some of the plants or shrubs that go around the home. After all, we choose what goes into our own gardens. Why should those living in nursing and residential homes not have the same choice? What about helping to weed? Most of us hate doing this, but for some people it is pleasurable. Just five minutes spent weeding, with thanks afterwards, can make a person feel valued. Raking over some earth that has been dug, or sweeping up, are both useful tasks that someone may be able to help with. In dementia care simply watching another person tending a garden is an obvious way of being involved. Picking a flower for someone to hold, touch or smell can give pleasure and enjoyment.

The domestic staff

Many of the older generation were particularly houseproud. The little carpet sweeper used to come out after every meal. Having a light carpet sweeper to hand presents an opportunity for a resident to offer help spontaneously and to feel useful. Giving someone a duster and letting him or her use it could give the same satisfaction. It does not matter how well the job is done. It is allowing a person to feel they have something to offer that is important. Most of us would hate to be in a situation where we felt that we had nothing to contribute. Cleaning brass is another task that many enjoy and this can be totally absorbing. There is a sense of real achievement in seeing a brass object newly cleaned and shining.

The chef

Having food that we choose to eat and enjoy is important to us all. When there are less busy times, the chef can discuss menus and try to talk to people individually about what they like. The chef needs to communicate on a regular basis with those for whom he is cooking. Sitting down and talking about food and sharing time enables the chef to be out of his rather isolated work environment, and to be part of the main body of a care home. Obviously there are many people who cannot articulate their likes and dislikes. Gaining information from relatives and care staff about likes and dislikes is vital. Helping to lay tables is an obvious area where people should be encouraged to help if they so wish.

The laundry assistant

Folding napkins or flannels, after washing and drying, is an uncomplicated, sedentary activity that can be done individually or as a group. This activity can be performed by anyone. We all fold the washing, fold sheets. There is something intrinsically satisfying, for many, in taking a basket of washing and creating order in folding.

The receptionist

A simple but extremely helpful task in homes where there is a lot of outgoing mail, is sticking stamps on envelopes. Helping to carry and put items of stationery into cupboards, and then taking away the empty boxes are also possibilities. These are tasks from which an active man could gain satisfaction.

There are also many tasks of daily living that do not fit into any particular job role. I recently visited a small residential home and on leaving noticed an elderly gentleman pushing a wheelie bin towards the house. I stopped to chat to him and discovered that he performed this task every week. He pushed the wheelie bins to the back of the house after they had been emptied by the refuse collectors. He was enormously proud of what he was doing in performing such a vital task. It was a valuable lesson to me in recognising the amount of creative thinking that is possible in relation to the tasks of daily living.

Self-occupation

The more able residents in care homes can, if they choose, pick up a book, read a newspaper or do a crossword or jigsaw puzzle. They can actively make choices. Most people however need someone to access the materials in order that they can occupy themselves. Mobility is key to self-occupation. I might be sitting in a chair unable to move because of my illness. My desire to do some embroidery and occupy myself would be dependent on someone talking to me, finding out what I wanted to do, and then bringing the silks and tapestry to me.

The activity coordinator and care staff are the people best suited to encourage and promote self-occupation, and both disciplines have opportunities to do this during the day. Making it possible for someone to be self-occupied is often linked to seizing the moment, realising an opportunity for someone to do something and acting immediately. Seeing someone with dementia twisting buttons and pulling at clothes shows a need for sensory stimulation involving touching and feeling, a need for exploration. If a home has activity blankets with different things sewn on and attached, these can be used to promote self-occupation. Buttons, ribbons, scarves, pieces of velvet, silk – all sorts of things can be used. How much better it is positively to engage someone in this way, than for staff repeatedly to have to pull down a lady's dress or prevent a resident from pulling buttons from a cardigan.

One very satisfying but simple way to encourage self-occupation, is to give someone a pencil and paper and thus encourage self-expression. I worked with a gentleman with severe dementia who, with tremendous concentration, would spend hours writing. He would repetitively fill part of a page with letters or crosses, and found his occupation totally absorbing. Another gentleman I knew had worked as a carpenter. Given a pencil, he would always put this behind his ear, then remove it and put it back again. When working, this was where he kept his pencil. This gentleman also enjoyed moving a ruler over paper, seemingly creating different angles. Then there was the resident who taught me to really look at artwork. He had been sitting sketching with a pencil and concentrating intently on the task in hand. When he had finished I asked rather tentatively what he had drawn. It looked amazing – fine pencil lines all over the page with lots of circular objects, all more or less the same size. I will never forget the withering look he gave me with the response, 'Melons large and ripe'. We should never underestimate the creative skills and imagination still latent in those who have dementia.

How much of a Challenge is it to bring Activities within the Remit of every Care Professional?

Care homes are busy places. There has to be routine and generally all staff have specific work to do. In the small home that I described where the gentleman enjoyed the task of bringing in the wheelie bins, the workforce is stable. Staff do a variety of different tasks. They deal with personal care, clean rooms and help in the kitchen. They do whatever is necessary and there is no demarcation of labour. There is no activity coordinator, but activity seems to happen naturally.

We learn about those in our care as we work. They are our teachers. A rapid turnover of staff disrupts this learning process and inhibits best practice. Whatever the size of the home, the potential for best practice exists where there are senior staff who understand and are keen to develop a culture of therapeutic care and a stable workforce. In many areas of the country there are difficulties with recruitment of staff for care homes. Given these problems, how do we then achieve the best practice in activity provision for those in our care, and how can the activity coordinator play an active and valued role? Input from all disciplines does, I believe, open doors to a lifestyle which actively promotes well being for residents, and potentially provides greater job satisfaction for staff.

Perhaps we should consider a new approach to the training of staff. If we look at the job descriptions of care staff they are geared generally to tasks. I believe that the title of care assistant should be altered to care activities assistant. This, in itself, would help to change the perception of what the role means. All care assistants need to have a period of training with the activity coordinator on a culture of care activities. It is so important that they understand the vital role they play in the well-being of each resident. We have to ask people to stand in the shoes of those they care for. We need to encourage new ideas and challenge thinking. Regular meetings between the activity coordinator and small groups of care staff could provide an opportunity for all to exchange views, feelings, thoughts and ideas. The activity coordinator does not have a monopoly on ideas for best practice, and ideas cannot develop unless all staff work as a team. Leading involves listening and learning from others.

In an ideal situation, the activity coordinator should complete assessments of the activity needs and abilities of all residents. Care staff should be aware of these assessments and should be actively using the information. There is little point in having activity assessments tucked away in a file unless they are regularly read and acted upon by other disciplines. The situation in homes where there are a large number of agency staff obviously makes things difficult. By the very nature of their work, agency staff tend to come and go. This is not to cast aspersions on the ability of agency staff, but a consistent body of staff is necessary for building support and understanding in any workplace. Perhaps we should be looking at encouraging agencies to set up professionally-led training programmes for their staff to encourage a culture of therapeutic activity. At present, the training on offer to agency staff often seems to concentrate on a task-driven work ethic. If the job title of the care assistant were to change to care activities assistant, then agencies would need to rethink the role fulfilled by those in their employ. It is clearly in the interests of all agencies in the care sector to provide well-trained staff.

Can unit managers, burdened by staffing problems and with large numbers of non-regular staff, realistically be expected to hold on to the ideal of a therapeutic activity culture? They have to try, because not to do so is to accept less than the best for those in their care. Senior staff, in conjunction with the activity coordinator, could develop an information pack on the activity culture which exists in the home. This could be used for new staff, agency staff, residents and relatives. Agency staff need a proper induction in any home. This may be time-consuming, but if it leads to a better understanding of what is expected of staff, then the benefits for all – residents and staff – must outweigh any difficulties. Care staff should be encouraged to support and help those who do not know the home as well as themselves. Respect and understanding towards all staff is key to a happy and successful home. A happy and successful home provides the best care.

If we go back 20 years or so, the idea of activities was just beginning to grow. Before then people in care homes were expected not to want anything other than their physical needs met. We all remember visiting places where residents simply sat around a room and, out of boredom, fell asleep. There was apathy, depression and tremendous sadness. People just waited to die. Activities then began to be introduced at a slow pace in some homes. Squares were knitted, basket weaving began its vogue and wood was sanded. Bingo made its entry and singsongs became popular. It was a start, and the concept of occupation for those in care homes began. At this time the culture of activity was almost entirely group orientated. The concept of occupation, in its broadest sense, was in its infancy. Activities had begun, but had a long way to go.

We now have a real understanding of what is required to bring a true activity culture of care to our homes. We have the knowledge, but have we the commitment and determination to push forward and change things? Changing established patterns and practices is not easy, but I believe that bringing all activities within the remit of every care professional is the way ahead. We limit opportunities for residents to benefit from the ideas and skills of others if one person alone is designated for the activities role. Job satisfaction has to be increased if all staff are encouraged to be involved in the activity life of the home.

To achieve the ideal towards which we should be working will take time. Every member of staff should have access to biographical details of residents. Without this knowledge, opportunities for occupation will be lost. All staff can seize the moment to engage residents in spontaneous activities and tasks of daily living. In a busy care setting the activity coordinator cannot be all things to all people all of the time. It makes sense for other staff to seize whatever opportunities may arise. This obviously requires a change of thinking, and an acceptance that breaking off from the task in hand and creating an opportunity for occupation is not shirking, but is part of the job. Clearly tasks have to be done and common sense has to prevail. I am not suggesting that the routine and smooth running of a home should be jeopardised, but that there should be a more flexible approach. Staff must be prepared to adapt, adjust and help one another. Job roles have to be seen as much more overlapping.

The role of a properly trained activity coordinator is pivotal to creating a new culture of therapeutic activity. This person should be training staff, coordinating ideas and leading structured activities. He or she should have the knowledge and understanding to follow up training, push ideas forward and inspire staff. Time should be spent with all staff, and meetings held which are totally multidisciplinary and about discussing ideas for activity, trying to resolve difficulties and talking about particular problems. While in most care settings there are regular staff meetings, these are often geared to groups of staff in a particular area of work. They are task-related meetings. Encouraging all staff to be involved in activity has the potential to raise morale and make people feel more valued.

Many may say that the ideal of activities as the responsibility of all staff is not realistic or practicable. To say this, and not to try, is tantamount to an acceptance of less than the best for those in our care. This is not an option. Nothing can be achieved without the will to change, a lot of hard work on the part of all staff and the desire to be at the forefront of best practice. I look forward to the day when occupation is so integral to the role of all disciplines that the activity coordinator role is not necessary. We have a long way to travel before that happens. Until then, we need many more trained activity coordinators whose contribution to the well-being of residents is properly understood and recognised to be as essential as that of nursing staff by unit managers and care providers alike.

CHAPTER 8

Providing Activities in Residential Care Settings: Dilemmas for Staff

Kenneth Hawes

SOCIAL AND THERAPEUTIC ACTIVITIES for older people have been a part of life in residential and nursing homes for many years, with many forms of activity being taken for granted and accepted as non-formalised aspects of the care environment. Indeed, we all recognise the value and importance that we place upon our own social and leisure needs, that is to say, they are basic human prerequisites. For example, staff and management at homes arrange day trips or outings for the residents, or traditional parties at Christmas and for other special occasions. These occasions are an integral part of the identity of care homes, not just within their own environment, but also within the local community. It can also be said that these events are often seen as opportunities for partnership, organised in a spirit of goodwill, with everyone involved adopting a role, thereby embracing residents, staff and management alike.

With the introduction of significant legislative changes during the 1980s through the Registered Homes Act of 1984, and the implementation of the Community Care and NHS Act since 1990, residential and nursing homes have become governed by principles of inspection and registration, and increasingly adhere to more formal procedures, advocating principles of accountability. In line with these changes over the past two decades, the role of the activities worker has gained increasing prominence within the health and social care professions. The position of activities worker was developed to meet this increasing emphasis on providing a more structured programme of activities for residents, and to enable the coordination of such activities with the other staff members and management of the home. In general, many activities workers come from a background of working in day centre settings, where the emphasis upon the benefits of therapeutic activities is well recognised, and structures the organisation and day-to-day running of the centre.

The importance of social and therapeutic activities is therefore now formally recognised within the guidelines that govern good working practices within the residential and nursing sector. This can be illustrated by its inclusion within care planning, whereby methods of meeting a person's needs are set out and agreed with the resident and, if applicable, their family member(s), key worker and home or residential care manager.

However, in some establishments the introduction of an activities worker has led to the responsibility for meeting all activity needs being transferred solely to that activities worker; in effect, creating a separate role to care, rather than the whole team taking responsibility for meeting a person's need. It is this dilemma that we set out to explore within this chapter.

Feelings about Providing Activities

The idea of providing an environment that promotes the value of activities within residential settings is one which most of us aspire to. However, many care staff do not feel that they have a responsibility to provide activities, or simply cannot provide them, due to the other demands of their working roles having to take priority; for example, attending to certain aspects of the daily routine, such as assisting residents with their personal care tasks. Factors such as staffing levels, practical support from management and general pressures of work therefore play a part in how committed we are about including activities within our daily programme of care. In many cases, the provision of therapeutic activities becomes an afterthought, and is given less consideration than other aspects of caring for people in these environments.

Who knows what care staff feel about providing activities? Does anyone ever ask them? Even with an activities worker in post, the responsibility for providing activities will, for the most part, fall on those who are involved in direct care with residents (ie, the staff members), due to the activities worker struggling to balance an average caseload of 40-plus residents and needing support. Hence care staff are required to perform this role alongside their everyday duties. This places greater pressure on them to balance their time more effectively, and the provision of activities joins the growing list of tasks the care staff are expected to perform. All too often care staff are not asked for their feelings and opinions as to how they can realistically achieve this goal. Consequently this can be considered by some staff members as more of a chore than an enjoyable and rewarding part of their work.

This is not to say that care staff do not enjoy providing activities. On the contrary, many staff would appreciate having more time to spend participating in activities, but often feel under too much pressure to cope with this extra responsibility. It would appear that little consultation has taken place with care staff about how the current situation could be improved and how to resolve these dilemmas. Indeed, it would also seem that the difficulties that many staff members face are not given adequate recognition, and these issues continue to be largely unaddressed.

In addition, some staff members feel uncomfortable providing activities as a formal part of their job. Where this is the case, there is a need for an increased understanding of what can be termed an activity;

that is to say, an acknowledgement that activities also relate to a number of low-key and one-to-one tasks, not just to larger group settings which can be all too daunting for many workers to face. Indeed, many staff undertake these low-key tasks without giving formal recognition to the fact that they are participating in valuable activities. This lack of awareness is an area which needs to be developed. One way of beginning to address this is through formal training, for example, a basic course which covers the recognition of everyday tasks as activities and demonstrates the importance of the practical and simple things that we can all do to meet residents' needs in more creative ways. Some ideas as to possible means of addressing such issues are listed later in this chapter under the heading 'Everyday Activities'.

The current political climate of new national standards for care is placing additional demands upon care staff to keep up with these developments and changes to the ways in which they work. In striving to improve the ways in which we care for older people in residential settings, many staff feel that their work has not been good enough and hence develop low self-esteem about their qualities as care workers. In this present state of flux with such significant changes taking place, the clarity of the care worker's role appears to have been somewhat obscured, which can only lead to confusion and frustration for the staff themselves. Clarity of purpose is a quintessential requirement in providing care in residential settings and makes addressing this issue even more vital:

> If a home is to run well everybody must know what it aims to do. There are many occasions when there are competing demands, in particular upon staff ... Of course without clarity of purpose it is impossible to evaluate the care provided. It is also vital to remember the ease with which a statement of purpose can be put aside. Like many other mission statements it can decorate the foyer without being related to practice. (Clough, 1999, p211)

Obstacles

Consideration of the emotive issues that are implicit within care work is essential in order fully to understand the implications of the ways in which care homes manage the provision of activities. It is necessary therefore to enquire a little further into the everyday difficulties and demands placed on staff providing the direct care to residents, difficulties that may prevent activities from being put on the agenda.

Stress

It cannot be denied that care staff have a difficult job to perform. They regularly work long hours, including weekends and bank holidays, as well as overtime, in order to make up their basic wage. Furthermore, it is a well-known fact that pay and conditions for staff in care homes are poor. The work that they do is physically and emotionally stressful, with workers balancing their time between personal care tasks, cleaning, assisting at meal times, doing laundry, etc, as well as caring for clients who may, for example, suffer from advanced dementia and/or whose physical frailty requires a high degree of manual handling and assistance.

In addition, other demands upon time and energy have gained increasing prominence over recent years, such as the emphasis upon the new care standards and the implications this has for increased accountability. On the one hand, care staff are expected to perform in a more skilled manner in their everyday duties, while on the other they often receive little guidance and support in their professional development and have inadequate access to supervision. It is therefore no surprise that care staff often feel undervalued.

Distance management

For the most part, this issue does not appear to have been successfully resolved at management level, and there are frequent problems faced by managers in 'getting the best' from care staff. Since the introduction of the

Community Care and NHS Act in 1990, there has been a shift in the running of residential and nursing homes towards a management culture, whereby the senior managers of a home have become increasingly distant and removed from the day-to-day running of the units. This style of organisation, based on the principles of the management model, is questionable as far as meeting the needs of staff and service users within residential and nursing settings is concerned.

This management culture would seem to have become integral within many homes, to the extent that managers are regularly not aware of what is happening with the day-to-day running of the home, the care of the residents and the working conditions which care staff face. It is rare for a management style such as this to adopt the principle that advocates managers taking a 'back to the floor' approach. Many managers of residential and nursing homes tend to have minimal contact with residents and, for example, would not consider participating in any basic personal care tasks. This has the danger of further perpetuating the divisions between care staff and managers, and can even be seen to set an underclass agenda.

More attention needs to be given to monitoring the style of management that exists in care settings. Staff members need more opportunities to be able to speak freely and confidentially with inspectors of homes, since management accountability can often be overlooked (for long periods) by routine methods of inspection. The idea of 'whistle blowing' on your superiors is still extremely difficult, and fear of reprisals is great. Inspectors of homes need to include sufficient time to speak to groups of staff about such concerns, since individuals generally do not have the confidence to speak their minds so freely. If staff are to give their views honestly, they must also know that they will be protected after inspection:

Bullying and harassment are very serious issues and so it is important that they are not 'brushed under the carpet', as they can be seen to be major sources of pressure, and therefore potentially of stress. (Thompson, 1999, p76)

Low professional esteem

If you mention to care staff the old joke about calling themselves 'bottom wipers', most will immediately relate to this. Care staff can feel this way because of the dilemmas and demands of their jobs, together with the manner in which they are often treated. Most professionals who are decision makers have long forgotten what this feels like. Some have never worked in a care worker role at all. If policy and practice are ever to run alongside each other and succeed, then senior decision makers must make time to 'return to the floor' with residents and care staff on a regular basis. Care staff require ongoing meaningful consultation with decision makers in order to feel supported by their management teams. If this cannot begin to be addressed, then 'bottom wipers' will remain the ongoing joke, and care workers will remain excluded.

Ethnic changes

It is also important to note the effect that changes in the ethnic composition and diversity of staff and resident groups have had upon residential settings. In more recent years, and especially within inner city and larger town settings, staff groups include many cultures in comparison to previously, when it was more typical to employ people from the local community. No one would dispute that we should encourage diversity from all areas, but we also need to help each other understand any community or cultural differences that may occur, in the hope of building a strong employee community in the workplace. This is an area that can be neglected within residential settings, thus forming barriers to working in harmony, with the consequence of creating a lack of belonging and an adverse effect on the community spirit of a care home. Without this community feeling we can feel distanced from each other, which can affect how we interact and how we organise events and activities within the home. This sense of community spirit is especially essential within the provision of activities, since many initiatives grow from feelings of belonging and goodwill. We also need to share our knowledge in order to relate to our client group and facilitate their relationship with us.

Training and Development

Despite the inclusion in the NVQ training programme of material relating to the importance of activities within residential settings for older people, it would appear that training in the provision of activities for care staff remains a low priority overall within training and development programmes.

Reminiscence training workshops probably come the nearest to some form of training in this area, since this therapeutic idea is fairly well accepted throughout the health and social care sector. However, this too is rarely given priority as an essential for care staff to undertake. Consequently it is not uncommon for care staff to know little about residents' earlier lives, or for residents to be encouraged to share their life experiences.

It is fair to say that there is a training need concerning basic activities awareness for both care staff and managers, in which the meaning of activities and what exactly can be described as an activity within a care establishment can be defined and explored in more depth. Even in the absence of formal training, people who supervise and manage homes need to take an active role in ensuring that staff gain an awareness of how to incorporate activities within their roles, and that they are supported in this within the constraints and demands of their primary daily duties. The concept of person-centred care is still in the early stages of implementation in many homes, and it is hoped that this will bring greater understanding of activities for daily living. Activities are as important as any other area of care provision, and a manager must ensure that staff will be supported in this new area until it becomes more comfortable and a regular element of their work.

Management teams have an enormous amount to gain from establishing a system of greater mutual respect and improving working relationships with care staff. Through their experience of working 'on the shop floor', care staff have practical ideas and everyday current knowledge about the residents they care for. Their experience and knowledge must be utilised since they have a lot to teach management at all levels on daily issues. Despite this being a key factor in unlocking many difficult areas of practice and thus leading to improving care standards, it can often remain a matter rarely given priority by those managing their units.

Documenting these areas in this fashion may seem a very harsh way of looking at care establishments. This is not to ignore the many residential and nursing homes that are working well in providing care of a very high standard and considering their staff in a fair manner. Rather, it serves to highlight my own observations after working as a care worker and activities worker over many years that, despite significant changes in legislation governing homes, the basic prerequisite of a person's occupational needs is still often overlooked in organising care in many establishments.

Everyday Activities

When we return to the question of providing activities, where do we start? If care staff are under such pressure every day, then how is it possible to consider activities alongside other duties? Furthermore, the realm of activity provision remains a rather vague and contentious issue for many managers and staff, with minor emphasis placed on the importance of a structured activities programme.

What can be realistic for staff, therefore, when it comes to providing activities in care homes? It appears there are enormous pressures that stand in the way of improving everyday standards, let alone the introduction of what may seem like another area of care to take into consideration. It is fair to deduce that unless some of the issues covered within this chapter are adequately addressed, the difficulties faced by many care staff are likely to continue to cause stress and frustration, and also to deprive residents of their basic needs. However, as professional care workers, we still have to persevere in the attempt to work to high standards in spite of these inherent problems.

Listed below are some areas that we can endeavour to include as activities within the day-to-day care of older people in residential and nursing settings. It is envisaged that these activities can be attempted alongside a care programme without too much extra demand on staff. All of the following are activities, and, although they may not generally be considered as such, they are just as important as any other form of activity. Some readers may recognise that these are regular everyday occurrences in their home. If so, then you are providing a very good foundation:

1 Choose appropriate films, television and radio programmes, news items and music and involve the residents in voicing their particular choices. There are suitable films most afternoons and some mornings in the television guide.
2 Provide a variety of newspapers, large print books and magazines. Local libraries will give advice and deliver regular book changes.
3 Arrange the unit environment for comfort and privacy with good accessibility for those with visual and hearing impairments.
4 Keepe the unit environment bright, clean, tidy, safe, accessible and decorated to a good standard.
5 Provide stimulating materials such as photographs, pictures, flowers, plants, a noticeboard, or reality orientation board with daily information written clearly for residents to be able to read.

6   Participate in general conversation with residents in groups and on an individual level, thereby encouraging them in social interaction on a day-to-day basis.

7   Create a relaxed, fun atmosphere by sharing snacks, drinks, fruit, etc with the residents as a separate activity from mealtimes.

8   Hold 'mini parties' to celebrate a special day and put up balloons and posters to mark it as an occasion. Consider inviting residents from other units or other parts of the home to come and join in with your unit's social time.

9   Escort residents out on a short walk/wheelchair trip within the local area, such as the park, local shops, around the block, or even to sit out in the garden whenever possible. In winter time a walk/wheelchair trip around the inside of the home can make someone's day.

10 Residents often spend several days during which they barely look out of a window and see the world outside, so, where possible, set up a seat by a window. Open the curtains in an area so residents can look outside.

11 Encourage visitors, volunteers and family members to feel welcome and comfortable by involving them in everyday life on the units.

12 Invite residents (if this can be achieved safely and under supervision if necessary) to help with tasks such as dusting, laying the table and washing up.

13 Hold residents' meetings. You may need help from other staff or managers to organise these meetings, but it is essential to try and listen to the views of the people who live in the care home on a regular basis.

14 Personal care tasks can be very therapeutic as an activity, such as spending quality time with residents when assisting with dressing, washing, shaving, bathing, cutting nails, doing make-up, styling hair, etc.

15 Smiles, laughter, warmth and friendliness with residents – a sense of humour and a good laugh can be one of the best activities of all.
16 Sing-alongs of favourite tunes can really change the atmosphere. Add a dance and a glass of sherry.
17 An activities box kept on the unit can include games, cards, quizzes, soft balls, arts and crafts materials, reminiscence photographs and objects and music tapes of well-known songs.
18 An activities timetable may help to initiate weekly times for certain activities. This time will need to be monitored by management or it may have a limited effect and become short-lived.

Although it cannot be denied that time can sometimes be a problem in arranging and organising activities, there are strategies that can be adopted to plan your day at work more effectively. For example, you may need to arrange certain activities in advance, and book some staff cover with your manager so that you can plan a particular social activity with your key clients or the unit. Key workers may wish to plan this in their supervision sessions.

Activity Worker's Role

There is much debate about the role of the activities worker within residential settings and how vital it really is. Is it more constructive to have a specialised activities worker or does this prevent care staff and management from assuming some responsibility for the provision of activities? This area is addressed in Chapter 7.

Because of the current dilemmas, it is difficult to determine whether it is more beneficial to have an activities worker who has a specialised knowledge and is able to concentrate solely upon this area of need, or whether the care team should be developed to work towards taking responsibility for all needs, including the provision of activities. The issues highlighted within this chapter illustrate the continuing obstacles to achieving a consistent approach to activity provision within residential and nursing homes. A somewhat idealised notion that activities can become incorporated as part of a daily routine which is undertaken as a common-sense and normalised approach remains at present difficult to envisage. It may seem convenient to pass the responsibility for providing activities to an activities worker as a role other staff do not have to consider. However, this contradicts the very nature of the holistic and person-centred perspectives on caring for older people.

Essentially, much of what we wish to see in the way of improvements for care and activity provision will ultimately be the responsibility of care workers to provide on a daily basis. It is clear that certain issues regarding the dilemmas and conditions for care staff working in these settings have not been adequately addressed, and this is hindering the achievement of higher quality care. As well as client-centred care, it would seem as necessary to develop a parallel policy of 'staff-centred' care. If we believe in the values of person-centred care for our residents, then we need to think a little more about who will be giving this person-centred care. If staff are able to work in appropriate environments and conditions, then it is likely that the residents' needs may be more fully met.

Person-Centred Care for Staff

The University of Keele Centre for Occupational Studies undertook an interesting research programme. From their conclusions, they developed a code of practice for staff care within health and social services.

The basis of a staff care policy is to provide an officially recognised holistic support network and procedures for the benefit of staff and management. This policy will endorse the principle that a healthy staff group performs its task more efficiently, and hence reduces organisational costs and waste, producing an overall improved quality of care: 'The concept of an external market for clients/customers needs to be matched by a concept of an internal market for staff, who are consumers of staff care and welfare provision. Employees who need help should, therefore, have choices' (University of Keele Centre for Occupational Studies, 1991).

According to the Keele study the provision of staff care has two components:

- *proactive* – directed at assisting employees to maintain good mental and physical health;
- *reactive* – directed at assisting employees to recover from mental distress or physical illness.

Proactive staff care includes education, training and assistance to develop good organisational practice towards employees. This may include awareness of stress issues, acquiring new coping skills and contributing towards organisational policy, practice and procedures regarding staff issues.

Reactive staff care includes provision of suitably qualified personnel to assist individuals or work groups who are experiencing problems to address their difficulties productively. This may take the form of confidential personal counselling or assistance from an independent team consultant.

There are other factors to consider that must be incorporated into an effective staff care policy:

1 Commitment to staff care at the highest levels of management;
2 Formalised workplace agreements with shared responsibility of all employees to sustain these agreements;
3 Recognition that line managers have limits to what they can do, hence the development of complementary support systems;
4 Training departments are a legitimate integral part of staff care provision;
5 All employees require training in the use of a staff care policy to explain its benefits and procedures;
6 Nominated staff care workers need specific training for this role;
7 Personnel to provide specialist staff;

8 Regular monitoring and evaluative research procedures need to be built into staff care at the planning stage.

In order fully to achieve the aims of adopting a person-centred approach for our client group, we must also adopt a policy of person-centred care for staff. To be successful, these approaches must complement each other, working side by side. A common sense stance advocates that if employees are happy, well organised, supported and valued, then care practices and the provision of activities should improve dramatically. Many of the difficulties commonly experienced are certainly manufactured from within the care home establishment and organisation itself.

Conclusion

This chapter is based on my personal experiences and observations through a number of years working alongside management and care staff within residential and nursing settings for older people. It has been written with a genuine passion to improve residential and nursing care for the residents, and for management and care staff to improve the effectiveness of their roles, thereby enhancing satisfaction with their work.

In some ways the chapter has presented a rather negative view of the current management structure of residential and nursing sectors, with what appears to be little acknowledgement of the daily pressures faced by managers of these settings. However, these issues are not addressed here, primarily because, for the most part, managers, by the very nature of their senior position, have considerable influence in the running of care homes and hence many opportunities for consultation with other colleagues. If this is not the case, then perhaps there is a need for further discussion to highlight management pressure. Care workers, on the contrary, generally play a much lesser role within decision-making processes at such a level and I feel their issues are under-represented:

> The style of leadership and management makes a dramatic impact on the life of the home. There is considerable potential to influence the lives of residents. There is also the accompanying responsibility for what happens ... Management has to create the forum in which people can recognise the complexity of the task, define the purpose and be free to air their concerns ... The manager must ask herself or himself 'What is this organisation here to do, and what is my part in it?' If the task is unclear, or if the task is found to be different at different levels or in different departments of the organisation, the service will deteriorate and the client will suffer. (Clough, 1999, pp206, 210–11)

Creating a friendly, supportive and healthy working and living environment does not depend on extra resources, nor does it take a new wave of restructure. It is about forming positive attitudes where energy, ideas and open mindedness can flourish. Establishing high quality care, activities and other aspects relating to the new care standards, can only be truly achieved if there are real improvements in the treatment of care staff.

I wish to thank Delyth Shaw for all her assistance in the discussion and editing of this chapter.

CHAPTER 9

Activity Training in the New Culture

Tessa Perrin

I PROVIDED A TRAINING COURSE some while ago for a large social services department. There was nothing unusual in that – there have been many such short courses in recent years. This one was a little different though, inasmuch as it triggered some new thinking for me around the matter of training people effectively. You can of course train people until the cows come home, and many of us do, but how much of that training is effective is a moot point. The perennial dilemma for the trainer is how to know whether what you are offering is actually training people effectively. Is the information imparted, received, retained and developed, and does the learning achieved actually make the trainee a better practitioner? Does it improve the quality of life of the trainee's client – for this is really the mark of an effective practitioner? This is a variable that is extremely difficult to measure with any degree of rigour and accuracy.

What most short course trainers do to obtain a measure is to rely on a written evaluation at the end of a course, which may give us an indication of how a course has been received, but is virtually useless as an indicator of lasting change. In order to try and engage with this problem in some measure, the course I referred to above (which concerned an occupational approach to working with dementia) required the participants to carry out and write up a workplace assignment. There were four days of classroom teaching, during which participants were to formulate a plan for putting a piece of new learning into operation in their own work setting. It could be anything of their choosing, provided it had a relevance to their own role and their own particular client group. They then had a couple of months to carry this out and write it up, at the end of which they were required to return for a half-day feedback session.

A small number of people failed to do the assignment and did not turn up to the feedback session, but overall I was surprised (and gratified) at the effort most participants had taken to get the most out of the task. At the feedback session all testified to the benefits of the workplace assignment, which for most had served to anchor the classroom teaching into the practice setting and took them yet further on, having elicited fresh realisations, raised different questions and encouraged new aspects of practice.

The question principally under discussion during the feedback session was how to pass this on, how to disseminate this information and encourage similar learning across a huge elder care department which was extremely unlikely to invest in more than one of these courses per year. The participant group was a mixed bunch, but most were from home care or day care and some were managers. The group was unequivocal in its view on three matters:

1 All elder care workers must have a basic training in cognitive impairment as it affects older people. Not all elder care workers work with cognitive impairment and some work with only one or two who are thus impaired. Nevertheless the group was emphatic that all must be able to recognise cognitive impairment, for it is increasingly common in care settings and staff must be adequately prepared. This

was a matter expressed most fervently by the home care workers who, although generally well supervised, are mostly working alone and cannot just pop down the corridor for advice in a crisis in the way that a residential or day care worker usually can. Group members considered that basic training should be mandatory in the way that manual handling training is now mandatory.

2 Some elder care workers in a team must be well-trained in specialist intervention, ie any team should have at least one member of staff with a special expertise in dealing with the kinds of problems engendered by cognitive impairments. It was considered imperative that any team should have a resident specialist.

3 Disseminating information in this area is too specialist to lend itself to the 'cascade' model of training. There is therefore a practical and economic difficulty in getting appropriate training to the large numbers of staff who comprise the average care team.

The issues highlighted on this course were specific to therapeutic activity and the person with dementia. Nevertheless, they are issues which are common to activity provision in general, and have led me to believe that those of us who are active in the education and training of older people have three key tasks before us:

- to train and equip specialists;
- to provide a career structure;
- to consider an alternative training model.

Specialists

Our first task is to train and equip specialists. The specialist, as I see it, is the master craftsman – highly skilled in interpersonal communication and the use of occupation as therapy. The analogy of the master craftsman is an illuminating one worthy of some reflection. The master craftsman is not usually an academic; he has not learned primarily from books or spent years in college. He has learned his craft over prolonged, and often laborious, work on the shopfloor. He has learned by emulating those with a greater expertise, by making his own mistakes, by using each tool again and again until it acts in his hands on materials exactly as he requires. Above all, he has learned because he has a passion for his craft. He wants to get it right, and he wants to be the best there is.

I find this a helpful picture of the kind of practitioner we require as a specialist in this field: a person passionate about his craft (in this case the achieving of health and well-being in his client through the therapeutic use of occupation), a person experienced in the care of older people, ready to listen, learn and make mistakes, and above all a person with the gritty determination to be the best it is possible to be.

There are such specialists about already. Sadly, they are not always recognised as specialists for they have no formal title, no proper 'profession', no governing body which officially recognises or rewards their specialism, no regulatory framework which is able to determine who may be permitted to call themselves a specialist and who may not (or to say why). These are people from every discipline who have learned their craft through many years on the 'shopfloor' of the older persons' care setting and who by good fortune have intuitively understood the role and value of occupation in healthcare.

However, I think it would be true to say that these specialists are few and far between, in national terms anyway. We are glad indeed for their commitment, for this is a field in which burnout is far from uncommon, but we need very many more if the ever-increasing need in our care settings is to be met. It is no longer good enough simply to trust to good fortune, to hope that the right people will be attracted to, and want to remain in, the work; nor is it good enough to expect existing specialists to continue unrecognised and ungoverned. We must, with some urgency, address the issue of establishing a suitable governing body and developing a coherent career structure. This is not the place to discuss the former. Suffice it to say that, at the time of writing, the National Association for Providers of Activities for Older People (NAPA) is in dialogue with the College of Occupational Therapists on this matter.

The development of a career structure has, I believe, begun. The creation of a Level 3 Vocationally Related Qualification, accredited in June 2002 (Certificate in Providing Therapeutic Activities for Older People – 6977), is the first step towards that career structure. This is an award written by NAPA and developed and accredited through City & Guilds. We believe that this award will equip activity providers with what they require to call themselves specialists in this field; that is, to act both as leaders and exemplars in the matter of activity provision in elder care settings. The award is not designed simply to provide practitioners with a range of practical skills in which they can engage their clients for the next year (although we hope that they will certainly go away with some). Primarily it is designed to enable the practitioner to lead and develop the activity culture in their workplace. This person needs the authority to guide and direct others in activity provision, and the skills which identify them to others as the master of their craft. These qualities cannot, strictly speaking, be delivered in the classroom of course. They are acquired as knowledge accumulates, as belief deepens, as passion drives and as confidence increases.

Nevertheless our hope is that the training which leads to this award will provide the fertile soil in which such qualities can develop and flourish. It is of little consequence that this person cannot paint, hates bingo and has no particular feeling for reminiscence. What is critical is that she recognises that this care assistant is good at painting and has the confidence to teach others; that this domestic goes to bingo twice a week, and wouldn't turn a hair at being asked to run a session for the clients; or that this volunteer has a particular interest in reminiscence and wants to extend his skills. Her key role is the identification and nurturing of these gifts and their incorporation into the activity culture of her care setting. She is not primarily a doer – she is an enabler, facilitator and coordinator.

The Guide to Good Practice in Therapeutic Activities for Older People (NAPA, forthcoming) proposes two key roles for any care setting concerned about best practice:

- the activity therapist or coordinator
- the activity organiser or provider

The Activity Therapist or Coordinator
This would be the specialist whose task is to act as leader and exemplar. My personal preference is for the term 'activity therapist', which stands apart from the plethora of other terms commonly used to describe the activity provider in the care setting. In my view, it correctly describes the person who uses activity therapeutically, ie to improve function and well-being.

However, it is a term that elicits some concern in professional circles, where the term therapist generally signifies an extended (three or four year) training of breadth and substance at degree level. There are issues for occupational therapists in the matter of eligibility for such a title and in a perceived confusion of roles. The College of Occupational Therapists has expressed a wish to the Health Professions Council (the regulatory body for professions allied to medicine) that the term activity used in combination with the word therapy or therapist be legally protected for the practice of the occupational therapy profession. This would mean that the term could not be used by anyone other than an occupational therapist or an occupational therapy associate.

This would leave those specialists discussed above with little option but to adopt the lesser title of activity coordinator, or some other term. Does it matter? I think it does, for the pivotal issue of the new culture is that activity is delivered as therapy, not as entertainment; that is, that activity is specifically intended and used to make people better. To adopt a title which fails to clarify this anchors us ever more firmly in the old culture and diminishes the status of the title-holder, with all which that entails. However, this is a difficult and complex issue which cannot be dealt with here, and which is going to take some years to bring to a satisfactory resolution.

The Activity Organiser or Provider

This would be a subordinate role responsible to the specialist, who is more of a doer, concerned with the actual delivery of activities. This person may well have a greater range of practical skills than the specialist, but does not have or want the leadership responsibilities required of the specialist. This person is essentially an activities support worker. It is unlikely that this role will have the emotive issues of title (discussed above) attached to it.

Our next step then towards a career structure for activity providers is the developing of an award for the activity support worker. One of the recurring themes in the consultation feedback NAPA received as the City & Guilds 6977 was being developed was just this: what about all those activity providers who do not want all the theoretical knowledge of the 6977, who might be unable to work to the demands of Level 3, who do not want leadership or organisational responsibility, but who just want to be good at delivering a range of activities? It is a pertinent question, for it is clear that the needs of this group are not currently being met.

Our response to that question within NAPA, is that a Level 2 award for this group must indeed be forthcoming, but we make no apologies for dealing with the Level 3 award first. We must first train leaders. In fact, if we are producing efficient leaders and strong exemplars who understand how to pass on their skills and knowledge using an apprenticeship model (see below), one could argue that there is no need for a Level 2 qualification. However, we recognise that units having this dual post set-up are very few and far between. Most units have only one post (if any) and that post holder simply may not want, or be able to deal with, a Level 3 qualification. There is, in addition, a need to recognise and formalise the contribution and role of this person, and there is probably no better way to do it than to create a specific award. Such an award would major on equipping the practitioner with a wide range of practical skills and the knowledge of how to impart those skills to the frail older person. Thus far NAPA has not had the resources to set the wheels in motion for a new award, but now that the 6977 is up and running we may be able to turn our attention in this direction.

Alternative Training Model

Our third task as educators lies, I believe, in considering an alternative model of training to that which has prevailed in recent years. In the last 30 years professional training has seen a greatly increased requirement for academic rigour in education, for college-based learning, for fast-track routes to paper qualification. The latter-day development of NVQ has served to redress the balance somewhat, anchoring the learning process in practice, in the workplace. As I have pondered not only the needs of the designated activity provider, but also the need of the whole care team to engage with the matter of activity provision (see Chapters 7 and 8), I have come to feel that both the college-based model and the NVQ model are inadequate for our purposes. Increasingly, I believe that the old-fashioned apprenticeship model of training has much to commend it. The notion of apprenticeship returns me to my original analogy of the specialist as master craftsman, for apprenticeship operates by linking the novice with the master, in the master's workshop, often over a prolonged period, in order to learn from beginning to end the intricacies of a craft. The apprentice first spends much time observing and absorbing. He then starts to work under the tutelage and close supervision of the master. As the master is satisfied with the student's progress, he is allowed to undertake work of greater complexity and intricacy, and monitoring is reduced. Only when the master is satisfied that his student's skills are approaching the calibre of his own is he released, let loose on the world and rewarded with his own title of master.

I believe that improving the health and well-being of older people through the therapeutic use of occupation *is* a craft, a creative work in the truest sense of the term, ie an engagement of one's own uniqueness with the materials of the surrounding environment, to bring to birth a tangible new product (Rogers, 1959). Our work is a craft, an engaging of all that we are – the unique mix of qualities and skills that identify and define us, with the unique mix of qualities and skills that identify and define our client, bringing to birth something new in that client through a consensual use of the therapeutic tools available to us. That 'something new' may be a new or renewed skill, a sense of purpose, a greater self-confidence, an increased self-esteem, a reduced anxiety, a manageable behaviour, a greater relaxation.

The work of using activity as therapy is probably unique among the healthcare professions, in that there are no standard procedures for practice. Medicine, nursing, physiotherapy and psychotherapy are all built around the use of standard procedures – for example, physical ministrations, exercise routines, modes of guidance – and therapeutic efficacy derives from these. By contrast, our work has few (if any) set procedures. Therapeutic efficacy ultimately derives from relationship, that is, the 'satisfactoriness' of the triangular relationship built between ourselves, our client and the tools/materials we work with. Therapeutic efficacy is crafted ultimately by you, the specialist, the instigator and the driving force of that relationship.

Relationship cannot be learned in a classroom or from a book. You cannot take an exam in it. It is, of course, learned over many years in the school of life. So if therapeutic efficacy is dependent upon relationship, our methods of education and training need to reflect that fact. Naturally some things may be learned in the classroom: basic psychology, knowledge of disabilities, analysis of occupations. But putting that knowledge into practice in the context of relationship with the client can only occur in the workplace. We need work-based training systems, and I believe that the apprenticeship model would serve us well in this matter. It can work very well in the context of care, with junior carers learning from, and modelling themselves upon, senior carers. However, in the care context, the majority of workers hold similar roles, and there is thus a ready-made 'workshop' situation. But this is not true (yet) of the activity context where any one unit is likely to have only one activity provider (if any at all). Currently the general older person's care setting does not lend itself to apprenticeship-style training, but that is not to say that we cannot work in this direction.

The responsibility for developing an apprenticeship model of training in a care setting would ultimately have to devolve upon the specialist. Providing that the specialist is sufficiently well-trained and experienced, there is no reason why this should not work. There would be two particular spin-offs from this for the care setting. First, they would be 'growing' their own specialists, who would be closely monitored and not released to work independently until a satisfactory level of competence had been demonstrated. The apprentice could quite legitimately complete the 6977 assessment process (workplace assignments and exam) without additional training courses, in order to acquire a paper qualification which would ratify their workplace competence. It is not inconceivable that organisations having multiple care settings would find this a cost-effective way of equipping an activity workforce, with monies being diverted away from less effective classroom-style training into financial enhancements for those specialists prepared to take on an apprentice. Organisations could adopt this model as a formal procedure.

The second spin-off of such a model for the care setting would be the informal acquisition of 'activity knowledge' by the rest of the care team. We have discussed elsewhere in this book the critical importance of all members of the care team engaging in the delivery of therapeutic activities. However a care team can really only learn from a model, who in this instance would not be offering a formal training, but who would be in a position to impart knowledge, to demonstrate excellence, to challenge attitudes and to shape practice.

Clearly we are asking a lot of this specialist. However, it is hard to see how we can really push best practice forward in the workplace unless this person drives it from the shop floor. As has already been mentioned, there are a goodly number of specialists out there already, many of whom are unrecognised and unrewarded. It is my belief that, if we are to move on, organisations must invest in the specialist in a way that has not thus far been addressed. Within an organisation, this person requires the status of junior management at the very least and a salary commensurate with that position. There are some activity coordinators who hold that kind of position, but they are very few and far between. So we press on.

I believe that the answer to the matter of training in therapeutic activities lies not in the creation of more and more courses, but first in a change of perception within organisations as to how learning occurs most efficiently, and second in an openness to adopting new models of training. We are going to need to see an organisational shift in attitude and practice regarding this matter if we are to move best practice into the future. Perhaps the responsibility for this lies primarily in the hands of NAPA, as the national spokesman for practitioners in this field. However, NAPA is only as strong and as skilled as its members. For those who are unfamiliar with NAPA, Simon Labbett gives an account in Chapter 14. The membership is growing and there is a solid core, but we would like to see a greater increase. There are those members who at membership renewal time choose not to renew, on the grounds that they 'do not get enough out of it' to warrant the £15 fee. In some measure one can understand this position. However, there is a view which suggests that one gets out of a thing what one puts into it, in equal measure. What NAPA critically needs at this point in its development are those who can 'put into it'. We need givers and we need fighters, for, without wishing to sound melodramatic, we have something of a battle on our hands. For all the changes that have taken place in recent years, for all that the new culture is beginning to make itself felt, the fact remains that activity provision in care settings for older people continues to be perceived as non-essential, particularly by resource providers. This is the fulcrum upon which the new culture will ultimately swing into its rightful place – when healthcare resource providers understand the critical link between occupation and health.

This is our task and this is the challenge to all those who really care about the matter of activity provision for older people: to build this body into a united front which can speak in high places with a voice of credibility, coherence and magnitude. It is a corporate task, but it is also an individual task. It is a task that really does need you. Please join with us.

CHAPTER 10

Activity Provision and Community Care: The Harlow Experience

Helen Crumpton

Merefield Day Centre

Harlow is a new town, built in the early 1950s, and has many of the problems facing other new towns of the time, including an increasing trend towards a predominantly elderly population. The large influx of people who moved to Harlow when the town was new and vibrant were in their twenties and thirties, coming with their families to get work and housing. The majority of these people never left, and this generation are now in their seventies and eighties, and need older people's services that were not necessarily planned for 50 years ago. It was estimated that in the year 2000 there were around 1,400 older people in Harlow with dementia or some form of mental health need. This is approximately 13 per cent of the retired population, yet there is a shortage of carers in the 40 to 65 age group, and dementia care services are in great demand.

Tom Kitwood (1997, p57) stated: 'Day care has developed in a very short time from being a type of 'minding' ... into a highly skilled and specialised form of practice.' Merefield Day Care Centre was set up nine years ago based on this modern attitude to care. It is a social-services-run specialist facility for older people with mental health needs. It is designed to be small and homely, but, because of this, it can only provide for ten elderly people a day, five days a week. Although this gives a high standard of care, there is great demand not only for more services, but also for a greater flexibility. In answer to this need, an Outreach Service was developed in May 2000.

Merefield's Outreach Service is based at Merefield Day Care Centre and has been built up from the knowledge and experience of the day centre staff. The Outreach Service is intended to take the day care that Merefield provides into the home environment. Kitwood (1997, p57) quoted Ely et al (1996) as saying that 'around 80% of all people with dementia are still living in their own homes; a substantial proportion – around 30% of these – are living alone'. Temporary funding was received from a government prevention grant to provide stimulation through a variety of activities, to help people who are socially isolated from becoming depressed, to prevent people from needing long-term care too soon, and to prevent a breakdown in their current situation. Merefield Day Care and Outreach are usually available to anyone in Harlow who is over age 65 and has some form of dementing illness or mental health need. Referrals have also been accepted for younger people with dementia. Most people are referred to the Outreach Service because, as well as their dementia, they are lonely or depressed, and the lack of stimulation is increasing the rate of the deterioration in their mental health.

To aid emergency intervention, it was arranged that referrals to the Outreach Service come directly to me as project coordinator. The referrals are usually received from the local Alzheimer's Society staff, the community psychiatric nurses, the social workers or from within the day centre itself. We limit access to prevent the service from being inundated, accepting only people with a confirmed mental health diagnosis. I then meet the referred person and their family and carry out an initial assessment of their needs. I arrange a regular time when an outreach worker can visit, then take one of my colleagues to introduce them, so they can visit regularly and build a one-to-one relationship. If a situation seems complicated or challenging, I will visit myself for a while, before introducing colleagues. With only a small number of staff, it is essential that at least I and one other member of staff get to know every client, so that we can rotate the visits to cover staff absences, ensuring that a familiar person is always available. The Outreach Service is focused towards people in four key situations:

1 Those who are on the waiting list for Merefield Day Centre when there are no vacancies. The Outreach scheme provides a few hours respite for the carer, and a few hours stimulation per week for the isolated individual until a place at day care becomes available. As one carer said, 'Mum is really looking forward to coming to Merefield and your visits are good preparation for her'.

2 Those who are waiting for social worker allocation, but are in need of some form of emergency input until a community care assessment can take place. An old age specialist at Harlow hospital commented on Merefield Outreach, 'It sounds like the stimulation at home is just what she needs'.

3 Those who are considering the possibility of receiving some form of care, but are not sure that day care would be appropriate. The Outreach worker goes into the home for a few visits to introduce the day care service and build up a trusting relationship, and later takes the individual into the day centre for a few hours as an introduction. One carer said, 'You have made such difference to her life. It is thanks to you that she is really going to start day care next week – this would never have been possible a year ago'. A social worker said of one of her clients, 'Congratulations on getting her to attend Merefield. She would not have even thought about it if she had not got to know and trust you at home. I never thought she'd accept any kind of day care, but she is enjoying it so much.'

4 Those who find that day care is not appropriate, either because they do not want to socialise and cannot deal with groups of people, or because they would find it physically exhausting to leave their home for any length of time. A carer commented, 'It is a unique and fantastic service that you provide; Dad is now too frail to attend Merefield and this gives us a much needed break. We all used to benefit from him visiting the day centre five days a week but you are able to provide an equivalent service in our home at a pace he can cope with.'

Visiting people who are socially unable to attend day care is an important aspect of the Outreach Service. They may demonstrate physically or verbally aggressive behaviour, they may become agitated in groups, or anxious if they are away from their home. Some people are uninhibited in their behaviour, and would not be able to mix with other clients. Because the Outreach staff have the training and experience to understand these people, they can be visited at home for one-to-one stimulation and care.

Willie was a sociable man who was keen to attend Merefield Day Centre. However, after a few visits he still did not seem to be settling. He became very agitated after a couple of hours, saying he needed to get out, and his daughter told us that he was quite distressed and tearful once he got home. After a lot of investigation and help from a local psychologist, it was discovered that the prisoner-of-war camp where Willie was held during the Second World War had the same layout of building as Merefield Day Centre. Although Willie liked the people, the experience of being in the centre was bringing back distressing memories. We started visiting Willie at home instead and he accepted the visits happily. Willie was able to join the day centre on a few outings so that he still got some company, but did not have to deal with the building.

The Outreach service provides a greater flexibility than traditional forms of care. For example, visits can be rearranged to fit in with appointments. Indeed, many times the Outreach workers have taken people for eye tests or to visit the nurse. It is also possible to offer the service at short notice or on occasional weekends to fit in with special plans, such as weddings, where the person with dementia would not be able to attend, but other members of the family need to. We have frequently provided a visiting service on bank holidays, as the person with dementia often does not know there is anything unusual about that day, or they have a greater need for the service if other facilities are closed.

We can do additional visits to cover family holidays, including evenings and weekends. Molly was cared for by her elderly brother. When he and his wife needed a holiday they were advised that Molly went into residential care for a week's respite. However, Molly did not settle in residential care, and when her brother returned home she was so upset and distressed that he decided he could not leave her again. Because the brother and his wife needed a break to be able to continue caring for Molly, Merefield were able to offer an alternative. Molly already received a home care visit each morning and evening and she attended Merefield Day Centre from Monday to Friday, but she was completely reliant on her brother at weekends. So, while Molly's brother was away, Merefield Outreach staff telephoned each morning to tell Molly what was happening that day and visited her as her brother would have done, carrying out exactly the same routine. On Saturdays we telephoned to say that we were visiting instead of her brother. We arrived at her flat at the time she expected him and took her to the same supermarket, then on to the same pub for lunch, then back to the flat at the same time. On Sundays we also continued the routine. This enabled Molly to stay in her own home and, as her brother said, 'This is the only way I could go on holiday and relax having the peace of mind that she would be well cared for.'

Communication and Building Relationships

Visiting people in their own homes on a one-to-one basis means that we build strong relationships in which people grow to trust us, and therefore we have some influence on most aspects of their lives. We can visit people for almost any purpose. Esther was not eating her 'Meals on Wheels' and was losing weight at a worrying rate, so we would visit twice a week at lunchtimes to encourage her to eat. We would take our sandwiches and eat lunch with her, making the mealtime a social occasion. After six months of visits, her daughter informed us that 'Mum's weight has stabilised and her iron levels are normal now and I am sure it is due to you visiting and encouraging her to eat.'

Grace had a stroke causing memory loss, severe anxiety and loss of mobility. When I first met her she was restricted to an upstairs room, kept in by a child's stair gate for her own safety. Her husband said he could not leave her alone in case she attempted to go down the stairs. In the past she had got part of the way down and had frozen with fear. The purpose of the Outreach visits were to give Grace some company as she spent a lot of her time alone upstairs, and to give her husband a break from his continuous care. The visits went well and, as Grace grew to trust us, she also grew in confidence. She would chat about many things and make jokes. We could encourage her to play dominoes or basic board games. She was still very anxious, but as her confidence grew, her mobility improved until she walked well around the upstairs of the house and became keen to attempt the stairs.

To encourage Grace to build her confidence and to help her regain some independence, we not only had to gain her trust, but also the trust of her husband. Understandably he was very protective of her, and worried that anything new or different might make her anxious. Having persuaded them both to allow Grace to try the stairs, they found she had the strength and confidence to get slowly, but safely, up and down them. The freedom of being able to sit in the lounge downstairs and to walk into the garden again gave Grace an enormous boost.

Once Grace was downstairs, it was possible to encourage her to go out of the house to a local coffee morning. Because she had grown to trust the Outreach staff, she would go with one of them each week, on the understanding that they would take responsibility for her. At her request, they would help her with access, mobility and conversation (as it had been a long while since she had socialised) so that she had nothing to worry about. Her husband again had to place his trust in the staff, since Grace had not been out of the house in a long time without panicking. She did not panic, and was noticeably more self-assured and confident when she was out of the house and socialising. Grace now goes out in the Outreach worker's car after the coffee morning, and has recently visited Merefield Day Centre and really enjoyed the company and activities.

It has taken nearly two years of visiting every week to build up the type of relationship in which Grace and her husband felt that they could trust us to this extent. By building up her confidence and abilities we were able to improve Grace's quality of life. To see the anxious lady who had been restricted to an upstairs room of her house now out socialising at the day centre is a great achievement for the Outreach staff.

Range of Activities Used

The most important and most basic tools that Merefield Outreach use to communicate and build relationships with people with dementia are conversation, music, books, magazines and photographs. They can be used as props or triggers for general activities, and can be subtle and not too demanding, but they are crucial in gaining trust.

Music

Music is an essential therapy for people with dementia. Most people have favourite tunes or happy memories brought on by music. People can be pacified by gentle background music or stimulated by the memories of good times. Many people with dementia who have little or no communication skills can still remember the words to songs from years ago.

Bert was described as having 'quite severe behavioural problems'. He was referred to Merefield Outreach by another professional who said she 'didn't know what to do with him' because he was a very agitated and restless man who found it difficult to interact with anyone. At the initial assessment visit I learnt, in conversation about his past, that he used to play the harmonica and had once played with Larry Adler. On our first visit we took with us a cassette of Larry Adler performing. Bert recognised it immediately and talked relatively coherently about it for a few minutes (to his wife's amazement). He would not usually let strangers stay in the house, due to his mistrust and anxiety, but we were accepted, perhaps because he recognised that we had made the effort to try to relate to him. On each visit Bert expected us to bring the cassette and, over time, we were able to introduce new music. Songs continually played quietly in the background and, although he still remained agitated and distressed, it seemed to be at a reduced level. There were moments when he would stop and listen to the music. Sometimes he would even sit down or sing along with the song that was playing. With prompting (while we followed him in circles around his house), he started to tell stories of how he would entertain the soldiers with his harmonica playing, and of some of the people he met while working in a London theatre after the war. The music provided enough distraction or reassurance to help Bert relax slightly, and it allowed him to think of the happy times he had enjoyed. It also allowed his wife the peace of mind to leave him with us for a couple of hours' respite.

Books and photographs

Josie suffers from dementia and severe depression. She is profoundly deaf and unable to leave the house alone, due to her lack of orientation. Although she lives with her daughter, the daughter needs to work full time to support them both. Because of this, Josie spends all her time alone and stays in bed, because she claims that she has nothing to get up for.

Due to her lack of short-term memory, she does not remember her visitors or the things that she and her daughter do together. She only seems to be aware of the monotony of being alone in the house.

When Josie's daughter is out, Josie cannot receive visitors because she cannot hear the doorbell or telephone to let them in. She often refuses to wear her hearing aid, saying that there is no point when she is on her own. Josie's daughter is rarely able to get her out of bed each morning, and she usually returns home from work to find Josie still there. Because Josie is not getting out of bed, she also is not eating or drinking enough, or taking her medication which could help to lift her out of this depression. She had also not left the house in months.

When I was contacted about providing Outreach visits for Josie, the main concern was how to get into the house to see her. We negotiated a lunchtime where her daughter could come home from work to encourage Josie to get out of bed in preparation for my visit, and then to let me into the house before going back to work. Initially this worked well, and Josie would get up, knowing there was a visitor coming. She would eat her breakfast with me present, and then we would chat or play games together. However, as the weeks went on, Josie started to refuse to get up for her daughter, complaining of pains or saying she was not feeling up to visitors. The daughter would allow me to go upstairs and encourage Josie to get up, but after a while she got used to me and I was greeted by comments such as 'Sorry dear, it was nice of you to come, but I don't feel like having company today – maybe another day', or slightly joking, sarcastic, comments such as 'Not you again, what do you want this time?' Fortunately Josie has a very good sense of humour and I was able to respond with a humorous comment.

I have learnt to take something with me to the house that could be of interest to Josie, usually a book or some photographs. I take it up to her room as a reason for visiting and say, 'I just called round to show you this.' After a while of trying not to look at what I have brought, curiosity gets the better of Josie and she sits up in bed so she can see and hear better. I usually ask Josie specific questions which encourage her to talk about the happiest times in her life. Although I have heard the stories many times before, I laugh along with her until her mood is lifted, and we can move onto other things. It has been known to take up to an hour of chatting, looking at books and general distraction for Josie to feel that there is something worth getting out of bed for.

Once out of bed, Josie will eat, take her medication and participate in any games or activities I have brought with me. By the time I leave she always says that she has thoroughly enjoyed the visit, and she looks forward to me coming again. Unfortunately, she does not remember this and we start anew the following week.

In recent weeks, however, there has been a remarkable turnaround. One day Josie's daughter was home from work sick, and, because of this, Josie was already getting up when I arrived. Once she was dressed, I said to her (as I had often done in the past), 'It is a beautiful day today, would you like to go out somewhere?' Amazingly, she said yes! The daughter told me not to get my hopes up as she would change her mind again, but I quickly found her coat and shoes and encouraged her out of the door. Once we were out, Josie was incredibly happy. She could not get over the flowers and trees in the park, and kept commenting how good the exercise was for her bad knee. We stayed out over an hour, to her daughter's delight, and when we returned she was able to tell her daughter much of what we had done. The following week she seemed to have remembered something of the trip out, but was still not keen to leave her bed. As the weeks have gone on, Josie needs less persuading and we have been going out every week. Her daughter has noticed that Josie is now getting up earlier each day and seems to be brighter. This week we even went to visit Merefield Day Centre. She said she really liked the atmosphere and would love to come regularly. This would be a great relief for her daughter to know that mum was safe in company all day.

Low-skill, high-reward activities

We have a lot of need for low-skill activities that still produce high rewards and provide a sense of purpose for people who have less ability, or are at the later stage of their illness. Music, looking at books with pictures and conversation are activities that two people can share at any level. In a similar way, dice games involve very little participation, just tipping up a container, but can produce much fun and reward when someone wins.

The initial reason for visiting Doris was because her husband was not able to leave her alone, and he needed a break to do his shopping. She was completely immobile and restricted to one upstairs room in the house. At this time she would call out and repeatedly ask where her husband was, even if he was in the room. She had a very short concentration span, and was easily agitated and distracted from whatever she was doing. The initial aim of the visit was just to provide the carer with some respite, as no one really believed that Doris would be able to improve, but we quickly noticed that she was starting to benefit from the stimulation.

By looking at family photographs, we started to build up a relationship so that she would trust us. Although she would call out continually for her husband, she would also say that she didn't mind us being there and liked the company. Her development (improvement) happened in stages, and we changed the activities, making them gradually harder as she learnt each new skill.

Initially we would take books to look at between conversations, particularly books with pictures that we could talk about together. Doris especially liked the royal family. These books would distract her very briefly, and she would begin to comment on clothes or hairstyles or her memories of the coronation. Over the weeks there would be longer periods of conversation and slightly less calling out for her husband.

We progressed to playing a game of dominoes where we would point to the dominoes Doris could use, and she would choose which one she wanted. She made no real attempt to move the piece herself and had no understanding of why she was doing it, but she had a willingness to identify the numbers.

As Doris became more willing to do things, we were able to encourage her to throw a dice and announce what number it was. This was her first physical participation, although still with no understanding as to why. She was able to participate in a variety of board games in this way. Later, Doris would move her piece around the board on basic games if encouraged, prompted and guided. At a similar time she developed the ability and willingness to put the dominoes she had chosen towards the centre of the playing area.

Nowadays, after visiting twice a week for the past few months, Doris is a changed woman. She is able to live downstairs. There is little or no distress and calling out. She has developed good conversational skills and rediscovered a great sense of humour. A recent stroke has left her with weakened hands, so she has less control when trying to move small objects, but she is still willing to try, and now she has an added determination. She enjoys a game of dominoes, participates fully and seems to understand what she is doing. She can play board games such as 'Snakes and Ladders' or 'Frustration' with little or no prompting, and has been known to explain the purpose of the game to her daughter when she visits. She enjoys large-piece jigsaw puzzles that she has been known to occupy herself with.

There seem to have been a variety of reasons for Doris' improvement, not least a sense of involvement from being downstairs again near her husband. He makes an effort to include her by wheeling her into the kitchen to dry the dishes while he washes them, or to peel a potato while he makes dinner. In the past, he would admit to leaving the room to get away from her, but now he enjoys sharing things again. He says that it is mainly due to seeing what she was capable of with a little encouragement during our visits. Initially the staff needed a lot of patience and perseverance to encourage Doris to participate in anything, but now, although she is still completely immobile and therefore inactive by some definitions, she is able to participate in and enjoy a variety of activities. There has been a dramatic improvement in her and her husband's quality of life. Doris' husband summed up his feelings about the Outreach Service when he said, 'I don't know how you've done it, but you've managed to work miracles with Doris. The time you spend with her is better than any pill'.

Carer's Expectations

Doris' carer changed his view of what her capabilities were after having seen how much she could do with our encouragement. The expectations of the carers often understate the potential. They tend to look at their relative as they used to be and say that (by comparison) they can now do nothing. Archibald (1990) said that 'So often we expect nothing and nothing is what we get'. However, carers are often surprised. The Outreach workers are taught always to focus on what the person *can* still do. According to Tom's wife, he had no concentration. She said all he could do was watch television and sleep. On Outreach visits she said I was welcome to try any activity that might be appropriate, but she warned me that he would not be able to participate. Tom is actually a very good dominoes player; it turned out he played years ago in the army. Chatting about his experiences as a child reminded him that he used to play and, with a little persuasion, he was willing to try again. Realising that he enjoyed it, he was then willing to learn a basic card game. His wife recently invested in a set of dominoes which he now plays with the grandchildren. She discovered that the card game I taught him is very similar to a game she plays with her friends, so one evening a week the television is turned off and Tom and his wife play cards together.

Fred had lost his powers of conversation and felt very frustrated by this, as well as quite useless because of his lack of ability to do things he used to be so good at. He often took his frustration out on the furniture since he was still physically quite fit, but couldn't express himself in other ways. It is increasingly believed that the type of aggression sometimes present in people with Alzheimer's 'is often the result of bewilderment and boredom. People need stimulation and occupation' (Campbell 1998). Merefield Day Care Centre, and later Merefield Outreach, invested in a magnetic dartboard. This enables full but safe participation in an adult game of darts, but with no risk from sharp points. It can be placed anywhere in a room to allow for varying strengths and abilities. It means that active people can have some physical exercise in a safe environment without risks. Fred's one great treasure was a darts trophy he won at a gentleman's club a few years earlier. However his wife would not let him play darts in the house in case he damaged anything (or himself). He had also been encouraged not to play in the local darts league any more. We were able to take the magnetic dartboard into the house, with his wife's permission, set it up on the sofa so that it was at a suitable height to be played from the seated position, and we would have a weekly darts tournament. Fred proved to be still a very good player. It gave him a sense of achievement and was a great surprise to his wife who thought he was no longer capable of anything.

Outings

Not only do we provide stimulation and activities within the home, but our service enables people the freedom to go out of their houses. Many people with mental health needs who live alone or with younger carers who work can feel very isolated. Either they cannot go out alone, or they may not find their way back if they do. Merefield Outreach is able to help these people to be less isolated and regain some of their independence. As many of them are very proud and feel they do not need anyone with them when they go out, we offer ourselves as a taxi service, while all the time befriending and chaperoning on activities that these people could no longer do alone.

Gwen has no family in this country. She can go out alone, but she likes the support, help with choosing clothes, or just the company itself since it gives her confidence and a feeling of independence. Ann has poor eyesight and cannot go out alone. Although her daughter does take her to the shops, Ann always considers herself a burden, and she feels rushed knowing that her daughter has other things to be doing. However hectic our lives may be, Merefield Outreach staff can, and must, always give the impression of having plenty of time for the people they visit.

Bill is a younger man with dementia who is physically fit and active. He lives at home with his wife. She still needs to work long hours to pay the mortgage. They moved to the Harlow area when Bill had to give up work, and he has not been allowed to drive since living there. Bill feels that this is the reason for his disorientation. He is not allowed to go out alone, and is always taken directly from place to place by his wife or a taxi, which has not given him the chance to familiarise himself with the town or to meet people. He is not only isolated, but feels that his independence and choices have been taken away from him. I visit once a week and allow Bill his own choice about what he wants to do that day. I have given him a map of the area where we are able to mark the places he has been, or where he wants to go. Often we just walk around the area he has chosen, commenting on the buildings and the people. Sometimes I have never been there either, so I can make it seem that we are navigating our walk together and I enlist his help to get us back to the car. Fortunately Bill realises that he could not go anywhere alone, but I provide him with the time to explore and become more familiar with his new environment. His map is his key to independence and record of achievement.

When I arrived one morning Bill was very upset. He showed me a card that his wife had given him that morning because it was their wedding anniversary. He was angry with himself because he had not known what day it was and was frustrated that he could still not make up for his oversight, since he did not know how to get to a shop. I suggested we to take a trip to town. Bill chose an anniversary card and, although it cost very little money, it had enormous significance for him and was a lovely surprise for his wife.

Intermediate Care

When I speak with carers they often comment that, as much as the stimulation is essential and the physical exercise a bonus, their relative also needs prompting with everyday household activities. As a family member, the carer often cannot discover what skills have been retained. Even simple tasks such as making a cup of tea are not always demonstrated in front of the carer, but this does not necessarily mean the skill has been lost.

A significant part of Merefield Outreach's role, particularly with people who live alone, is intermediate care. However, because our main aim is to keep a good relationship and be a trusted friend, persuading people to do household tasks needs to be done in a way that makes the activities enjoyable.

We have to be careful who we encourage with household activities and what we do. Iris has a habit of washing the electric kettle and has ruined many a kettle while soaking it. Her cooker is already disconnected for safety reasons, and home carers come in each day to provide food and drink at regular intervals. It would be inappropriate and potentially dangerous to try to encourage Iris to make herself a cup of tea. However, Iris is very house proud, so we wash up with her, wipe down the surfaces and help her to tidy the tins in the cupboards.

Nellie lives alone. She receives 'Meals on Wheels' each day and, until recently, she had very little ability to do anything for herself. However Nellie has been taking an Alzheimer's drug for the past six months and she is one of the fortunate people who has shown signs of improvement. She appears to have the ability to recover lost skills and I visit once a week, not only to help maintain the skills that still remain, but also to try to encourage the return of others. Nellie's main love was cooking. The first thing we were able to do together was stew some plums at her son's request. Under supervision and with encouragement, Nellie was able to prepare the fruit, find the saucepan, add the right amount of sugar and turn on the hob safely. As the plums were cooking it became apparent that Nellie had no concept of the heat of the cooking. First she tried to put her finger into the boiling saucepan, and then tried to taste the juice straight out of the hot pan. We later cut rhubarb from the garden and made a crumble. Again Nellie retained the ability to get a perfect consistency for the crumble, but any sense of the heat coming from the oven was lost. Later we made a sponge cake for her sister's visit. She was able to do all the preparation with only a little prompting, but agreed that I dealt with the oven and anything hot.

Nellie had not only lost the ability to cook, but also the confidence to try. With someone there to support and encourage, but not take over, Nellie found she was able to do a lot more than either she or her family imagined. 'Mum was so proud of herself for stewing those plums. She hasn't done anything like that in ages.' Nellie and I now have a safe weekly cooking session where she teaches me many of the tricks of the trade and I safely negotiate anything hot or potentially dangerous. Other than on this day, Nellie no longer cooks.

Success of Merefield's Outreach Service

Merefield's Outreach Service has had a significant effect on many people's lives. The people with dementia, their carers and their families have all expressed how much their quality of life has been improved by a service that takes day care activities into an individual's safe and reassuring home environment. It is a flexible service that is able to provide full support to older people with mental health needs while still encouraging independence. We are giving people confidence and hope by focusing on the positive aspects of their lives. Because the Outreach provides a flexible service to people who might not otherwise accept or be suitable for traditional forms of care, it has helped the whole community. Social workers, community psychiatric nurses and other community care workers have all praised the way in which the Outreach workers have been able to encourage people who have always refused assistance in the past into receiving services of some kind. The additional facility in Harlow also helped to reduce the waiting lists of other services.

I believe that the Outreach Service has been so successful because it was developed from an already established mental health day centre, using the knowledge and experience of the trained staff, along with the facilities and reputation of the centre. The Outreach staff have been well trained and are willing to be flexible to cover occasional weekends or bank holidays to help families for special occasions or emergencies. Rotas are also flexible to allow the Outreach staff to accompany clients to appointments. We are able to use the trained staff in the day centre to cover absence for leave or sickness and, equally, the Outreach staff have been known to help out when the day centre is short-staffed. This means that a high quality service can be provided at all times.

The Outreach Service shares and has extended the support network already set up by the day centre. This includes monthly troubleshooting sessions with the local older people's psychologist with whom we can talk in confidence to gain professional advice about specific clients. Outreach makes use of an already established direct link to the psychiatric services to help with emergencies. We have been able to maintain and expand essential relationships with the local community through Merefield's advisory group that meets to discuss the needs of older people with mental health needs in the Harlow area. The members include not only staff from the day centre and Outreach Service, but also local psychologists, psychiatrists, psychiatric nurses, GPs, social workers, Alzheimer's Society staff, carers and ex-carers, with occasional visits from local councillors. Harlow is very fortunate to have this community support network. It helps to ensure that people with dementia can have a streamlined service through each stage of their illness.

Cost Effectiveness

The Outreach Service has proved to be a very cost-effective way of caring for older people with mental health needs. Over the first two years (the first year with 48.5 staffing hours and the second year with 104 staffing hours per week) Merefield's Outreach project received almost 100 referrals. The three members of staff between them carried out over 1,400 visits, supporting over 80 clients and their families. Although each visit is only for a few hours, the three staff currently provide intensive one-to-one stimulation for around 30 clients. Because the service is intrinsically linked to Merefield Day Centre, it does not add much to the everyday cost of running the ten-place day care facility. The Outreach Service shares one office and uses the stationery and materials of the day centre. The main expenses are the staff's pay and mileage, plus the mobile phones that are an essential part of the Outreach; not only for the safety of staff and clients, but also for when a client does not hear, or will not answer, the door, and we use the mobile phone to tell them we are on the doorstep. Beyond that there are very few costs. Because we are in people's own homes there are no overheads for renting buildings or paying utility bills. The funding costs for the first year were only £17,750 for two part-time staff, increasing to £37,730 for the second year for two full-time and one part-time staff members.

We have had such positive feedback that the reputation of the service has spread across the county, and we are regularly being asked to visit people outside the Harlow area. Unfortunately the scheme has fallen victim of its own success, because we constantly have a waiting list for new people wanting the service. However, we are currently hoping to hear that the existing staffing posts will be made permanent and, at the same time, we have the promise of additional staff so that we can extend the service both within Harlow and to other parts of Essex.

Merefield's Outreach Service has changed people's lives. As the local psychologist said, 'The Outreach service has provided a good standard of intermediate care, preventing a lot of hospital admissions.' Joe's carer expressed the feelings of many others when she said, 'Merefield Outreach has been our lifeline this past year.'

CHAPTER 11

Activity Provision and Community Care: The Leicester Experience

Caroline Ryder-Jones, Wendy Ferguson and Rebecca Colledge

WE WOULD ALL WELCOME A WORLD where people with dementia have a full life, where they enjoy the things that are important to them and maintain a sense of purpose, routine, spontaneity and creativity. These things contribute to our overall sense of well-being. For one person, folding the laundry on a Monday is a vital part of their day. Another is absorbed with pricking out seedlings and watering pots of flowers. Both these things can be facilitated, whether a person is in a formal care setting or their own home. The challenge is to discover what is right for individuals and to determine a way of supporting them in pursuing that special something. This chapter aims to share why and how occupational therapists in Community Mental Health Teams (CMHTs) in Leicestershire started to address these needs; to explore the journey undertaken by us to change our style of work, and to discuss the process of assessment and provision, illustrating this with case studies.

The Background

Within Leicestershire, occupational therapists (OTs) have been established in CMHTs since 1991, with the OT service providing both OT-specific assessments and a key-working role. In practice, OTs were largely used initially as key workers providing a generic role. This meant we were mostly coordinating care, rather than providing OT interventions. Whenever a specific OT assessment was requested, it was generally for physically-based needs: a bath board, a stair rail, a raised toilet seat or a commode. At times we would provide an assessment regarding a person's ability to cook or get dressed; however, often these assessments would simply lead to a home care package. When, as a service, we needed to produce a document about our core business and place within the Trust, many soul-searching questions were raised. What was the core business of the OTs and what was the theoretical underpinning for it? What did occupational therapy provide that no one else did?

At around the same time we were reading work by the psychologists Tom Kitwood and Graham Stokes. They wrote of the person with dementia as a person with more than the simple physical need to be fed and watered within a safe environment. They recognised other needs, such as a person's need for purpose and emotional contact, and wrote of the effect that meaningful and purposeful occupation could have on a person's sense of well-being. We recognised these needs and felt we should be addressing them, but were unsure how to proceed. It was at this point that our journey first began as we started to try to address people's occupational needs in order to engage with them in a personally meaningful way. This involved exploring the human need for social, leisure and work roles.

The Journey

We started to explore this, and felt that some sort of assessment was required, but could discover none which were specifically tailored for people with dementia. We therefore devised a homemade assessment pack comprising: scissors and shapes to cut out; a pack of cards; some scented pots; a small jigsaw; and some dominoes. This was used to identify a person's ability to concentrate, follow instructions, sequence actions, recognise objects and to provide some insight into their memory function. This was useful in starting to explore people's skill level relating to activity, though it had limitations and these abilities were better assessed using other tools, which are discussed later. We recognised that in order to pursue this kind of work appropriate referrals were needed. For this reason, a team presentation was done explaining the link between engaging in meaningful activity and maintaining a sense of well-being. Then the role of OT and the way it could address the occupational needs of people with dementia was discussed. From this, referrals gradually trickled in. More OTs in the service became involved in the same role and the hard work really began. We could identify people's abilities and preferences, but then needed to match them up to enable people to re-engage with the occupations/activities they had lost and which their carers often saw as either impossible or irrelevant.

Over time the assessment process was refined. Better tools helped to identify the right type and level of activity for people. Evaluation methods were used to establish whether what was offered had any benefits for people with dementia. Experience helped to generate more ideas and increased confidence. As more work was done in this area, it was realised that the needs met by activities were about so much more than simply leisure in the form of playing games or pursuing a hobby, although this aspect was the one we had often focused on initially. The needs addressed related to the desire for a sense of role and purpose within their daily life. This work was about meeting a person's need for occupation in a wider sense, which would also include their day-to-day activities: from getting dressed, to when they thought the laundry should be done; from what they liked to talk about, to when they thought it was appropriate to go for a walk or watch television. The work needed to recognise each individual's life story, and the way it influenced their behaviour and needs. It must utilise activities that relate to a person's values and have a specific meaning for them. This became the focus of our OT service. The feedback we received excited and spurred us on. Two clients in particular impressed upon us the importance of knowing a person's life story.

The Major lived in a nursing home and, following intervention, I gave feedback to the staff in order to increase their understanding of him, and to facilitate their continuing appropriate occupations. He had been a major in the army and this had shaped his habits regarding the way he laid out his grooming tools and the military precision with which he made his bed. He had always been a charmer and had held a reputation as an international playboy in his youth. He often laughed about this, stating he probably had children in every country! He had enjoyed a privileged lifestyle and had loved driving fast cars, losing his driving licence three times for speeding. He had pictures from his days of wild parties and even a newspaper cutting describing how he lost thousands in a single game of cards. For the Major, it was imperative that he always had a carnation in his buttonhole and a newspaper in his hand. The thought of not wearing a tie or opening the door for a lady was abhorrent. He enjoyed a constitutional walk each morning and a sherry with his meals. These things gave him a sense of normality. He was anything but the stereotype people often have of the over sixties. When feeding this back to his main worker, she reflected how useful it had been, noting that she normally only found out such details during a person's eulogy at their funeral.

How sad that the very things that shape us are often ignored. Addressing this and finding out a person's life history can spur us on to reach out to people and give us the vital connection we need. This was further illustrated when working with Martha.

Martha had had a difficult life bringing up her four children single-handed, as her husband was an alcoholic and rarely around. She worked hard in a hosiery factory and came home to look after the children and keep the house in good running order. The concept of leisure time was foreign to her; the nearest thing to it being knitting clothes for her children, though out of necessity rather than pleasure. Staff had expressed concern that she frequently tried to leave the residential home, stating she needed to get back to her children and didn't have time to be sitting around. For her sense of well-being, she needed staff to involve her in the household chores. She was happy to have a duster in her hand and a tin of polish. She loved her carpet sweeper and most mornings she would be involved in doing dishes and peeling vegetables, or at least spending time in the kitchen amidst the hustle and bustle of activity. During the afternoon she was often found folding laundry. Her attempts to go home reduced, and on several occasions she happily told her visiting sister that she couldn't chat for long, as there was so much to do!

The Assessment Process

The assessment process we used involved gathering information about people's abilities and preferences. Initially, gathering information can seem daunting, as each person has a wealth of personal history and many different abilities. We often found it hard to know where to start when assessing for activities, so we used various techniques to help us through the process.

Gathering details regarding a person's history was vital. Initially we spent time talking to the person with dementia. We also spoke to relatives, friends, or carers who were very involved in the life of the person we were working with. Observation of people completing activities of daily living such as eating, dressing, chatting and so on, was essential to gain an initial idea of what they were able to do and to identify anything they found difficult. It also gave us an idea of what motivated that person to engage in activities. An awareness of the individual's interests was equally invaluable. We devised a leisure interest checklist (Appendix, p183), a questionnaire to focus discussion. It explored past, present and possible future activities that the person might consider, covering themes such as:

- Recreations – games, art, reading
- Hobbies – gardening, crafts, dancing
- Holidays – day trips, favourite type of destination
- Entertainment – television, videos, music, clubs
- Volunteering and education – group membership, church leadership, clubs, evening classes

The leisure interest checklist can be used in any setting to stimulate discussion about potential activities and can make things easier than starting with a blank sheet. It should highlight what to avoid as well as what to try. It also gives a picture of the client before they were experiencing their current difficulties, and becomes a reference point when fresh ideas are needed in the future.

An assessment called Pool's Activity Levels (PAL) (Pool, 2002) was also useful in helping us to pitch activities at the right level. It is an assessment tool developed by an OT and provided a more structured format for our observation. It uses information about what people can do or what they may find difficult when carrying out daily living tasks such as eating, dressing and communicating. This information is recorded on a checklist that gives guidelines by which activities can be planned. It is observational and not intrusive. It collects information in a straightforward way, and provides clear guidelines for formal and informal carers. We found it ideal for group settings such as day care and residential homes.

All of the above helped us to grade activities to suit different people's abilities in order that they could achieve success and fulfilment. A simple method for grading activities to match a person's abilities involves using an orange. A person may cut it up with other fruit and make it into a fruit salad, or simply peel and eat it. If a person is unable to manage that, the orange can be used as a sensory tool and they, or a carer, can push cloves into its surface and its scent can be enjoyed. Just as different levels of activities can be generated with an orange, the same principle can be applied to many other materials/activities. The key is to enable a person to experience a sense of achievement and/or enjoyment. Given that some people prefer to iron, some prefer to garden, some sing, some love sport, etc, the possibilities for experiencing activity are endless, and often only really limited by the narrowness of our imaginations and our own preconceived ideas about illness and ageing.

Experiencing the Activity

Below are examples of how we implemented programmes of meaningful activities with people with dementia.

Shirley had previously loved to cycle. This didn't necessarily fit in with the stereotypical view of a 76-year-old person with dementia, but she was fit and able and why shouldn't she continue to cycle if she wished? So we got on our bikes to ride, assessing her orientation around the village and her safety on the road, and now she regularly cycles through her village to visit her sister, providing her with valuable social contact and her husband with much desired space.

It was often important to involve carers in the sessions to provide the ideas required or encouragement needed to enable them to initiate such activities themselves.

Grace lived with her daughter's family. She was kept in an upstairs room and didn't come out as her daughter couldn't cope with her incontinence. Grace was a person with dementia, she was depressed, blind and her mobility was poor. She wasn't used to company and didn't tolerate visitors well. In an attempt to encourage her daughter to more actively meet some of her need for occupation and provide some ideas, activity sessions were instigated. She had previously enjoyed music and dancing, and therefore one session consisted of using a tape recorder, some music hall songs and percussion instruments. We sat in her bedroom singing and playing at the top of our voices. It was a simple, straightforward activity that was carried out amidst her daughter's scepticism and within an environment that was not ideal, but it created a moment when the activity briefly superseded all her difficulties. She delved into her memory for words to songs and surrounded us with noise. She showed great delight and she was truly engaged.

Even with encouragement, it was not always easy or possible to get carers on board. Some carers found it emotionally impossible; some had not previously had a relationship that involved sharing activities together. Some found it just too difficult to carry out activities for pleasure when they were tired out by the many challenges of providing day-to-day care. We found that it was sometimes more successful to link in with relatives other than the main carer – possibly grandchildren, friends, activity organisers or volunteers – with advice to assist them successfully to provide more long-term intervention than we, as OTs, were able to give. This was because, realistically, OTs were only able to provide assessments and short-term sessions and pass on information for others to utilise.

Hazel was a 55-year-old-lady who had a diagnosis of Alzheimer's type dementia. She lived with her husband who went out to work each afternoon until mid-evening. Hazel was left alone for that time, but sometimes became agitated and started to scratch at her hands, making them bleed. It was thought that some activity might help the situation. An activity assessment was carried out and her functional level identified that she was able to do activities which were based on repetitive actions like sticking and stamping, but that she also took pleasure in producing something to show her family. One of the activities identified on her Leisure Interest Checklist was that she had been skilled at embroidery and knitting. An activity session was organised, based on a very simple tapestry cloth with large holes, thick wool and a large, clear outline. During the session it soon became clear that Hazel could not independently initiate any action, requiring demonstrations and many simple verbal prompts. Although she attempted to sew the outline, she could not follow the motif. She became aware of this and made negative comments. The session needed to be adapted and, using the materials available, we changed direction and produced something she was happy with. The wool was used with cut-out cardboard circles and Hazel, with demonstrations and constant prompting, repetitively wound the wool around the cardboard to make a pom-pom for her small grandson. She enjoyed the process of 'doing' and appreciated having an end product. This was demonstrated by her repeated wish to show her family what she had made.

In this case, the original activity was familiar to Hazel, based on an activity that she had enjoyed and which had been simplified. It still did not match Hazel's abilities and the activity had to be adapted using the materials available during the session. Having then observed Hazel's abilities during that session, the observational information along with the assessment were vital in getting future sessions just right. We focused on repetitive actions and single-word instructions alongside visual demonstration or physical guidance. We used activities such as paint stamping to make cards and decorate wrapping paper, and simple glass painting on acetates, using large bold designs and brightly coloured paint. We also made scones which she identified as being a particular favourite, an activity which involved Hazel mixing and kneading. She did like to have something to show for her efforts and to present to her family and she enjoyed the company, despite her conversation being very limited. Five different activity sessions were completed, and then joint visits were arranged with a worker from a respite care service who, with the information provided, then spent afternoons with Hazel, sharing an activity during that time.

Often, having something to share with, or show to, others, provides an opportunity for people to give positive feedback, rather than pointing out what a person cannot do. Some people with dementia are able to take pleasure in remembering what they have done when they see it again.

Bindu was an Asian lady who lived with her husband. Since she was diagnosed with an Alzheimer-type dementia, her husband had gradually taken over all household tasks. She subsequently expressed feelings of boredom and had become tired and lethargic. She could not understand why she was no longer allowed to cook. She had also helped in their corner shop, but she was no longer thought to be reliable, particularly when handling money. Like many Asian women, Bindu saw her role within the home as looking after her husband, particularly cooking the meals and contributing to the household in general. Her husband felt she was no longer safe when using the cooker, and she could only make chapattis under his supervision. We identified and practised some straightforward dishes to make, and a worker from the respite care service visited some mornings and provided the supervision required while Bindu cooked. Thus she contributed to the household meal and regained some of her role. It was also fun for Bindu, who passed on her specific knowledge of Asian cookery to the worker, which enabled her to feel valued and more confident. Her husband was able to concentrate on running the business without the need to supervise Bindu.

During one of the cookery sessions Bindu spontaneously decided that she wanted to grow flowers. We shopped together at the garden centre, and she was able to make choices about what to buy. We spent a morning sowing seeds, which she then nurtured to finally produce her flowers. This gave her something within the home that she identified as belonging to her. She showed great delight on every subsequent visit in showing how the seedlings were progressing. I hadn't previously seen her so animated and excited.

As we have developed our practice in the area of activity provision in the community, we have been continually reminded that it is essential to enhancing the well-being of clients. They have often lost so much: their sense of identity; their roles within the home; sometimes loving relationships too. To be involved in something familiar can bring back a sense of identity and facilitate feelings of achievement, enjoyment and fulfilment that are invaluable.

In order to achieve this, it took a great deal of encouragement and perseverance on behalf of the people we worked with and the OT. Constant evaluation was required to make sure the sessions were achieving their aim, and we used the well-being/ill-being recording forms (Bruce, 2000) to map which activities created the best signs of well-being and which, perhaps, did not. Activities that were tried did not always work; the occasion when we tried hand massage with a lady who didn't like the smell of the hand cream immediately comes to mind. However, it was important not to give up, but to try a different approach, adapt to a different level of function, or consider an alternative.

Brian was a gentleman with a vascular dementia. This greatly affected his ability to communicate with others using expressive language. He had previously been a very active man, participating in various leisure and social activities. Unfortunately, he now tended to isolate himself. He had stopped activities he previously enjoyed and avoided social events, particularly family gatherings. Brian's family was keen to know how to help him. Brian had a great love of old movies, which was evident from his extensive video collection. Initially, the activity chosen was looking through a movie book, which mainly contained pictures. He seemed to enjoy picking out his favourite actors and films. This activity progressed to Brian watching a favourite film that was familiar to him. He enjoyed singing and dancing to the musicals. Brian's family became involved in reminiscing with him about his life. They used old photographs and made a life history book which helped Brian name dates, times and details of events. All of these activities placed less pressure on Brian to express himself through language alone and helped him to communicate with his family again.

Personal Thoughts

In many ways the above account sounds like an easy transition and is too simplistic. In reality, it happened over a period of approximately two years and was sometimes difficult and painful. At times we were unsure of ourselves, recognising we had a lot to learn and lacking the courage of our convictions. We were often challenged and had to justify why we were spending time on seemingly nice things, such as pleasurable activities/occupations, when there were so many other needs, such as organising home care/monitoring medication. In a sense, we were at times perceived as putting the icing on the cake, rather than making the next cake, and we needed to remain firm in the belief that what we were providing addressed quality of life issues, which are as vital a part of dementia care as the practical side of personal care. Some OTs, particularly those with a strong history of working in physical settings, struggled with the concept of addressing occupational needs and initially felt resistant to changes in the focus of our work. It is a terrible admission that at times, despite being occupational therapists, we debated whether we needed to address occupational needs.

Alongside the theoretical difficulties there were also practical ones. One of the problems of working alone within the community was that we did not have a bank of equipment/materials to hand, or a budget directly available for such things; although luckily some families would buy items on request when we knew that the item could be utilised with success. Familiar activities could be carried out using items available within the home, but often it was necessary to take materials along, and these were frequently borrowed or donated by our unit-based departments, or we had to go shopping. We found this type of work more time consuming, because of the need to travel to the units for equipment/materials, visit the shops, or plan the sessions. This was not reflected in our statistical data, which collects details of face-to-face contacts only. As this type of work was not seen as high priority, although it was valued, it was always hard to justify the time it took when we were short staffed.

Key factors that helped the service move forward were: the management structure; a team spirit; peer supervision; theories and research on dementia, such as that done by Kitwood and Stokes; occupational science; and the promotion of the role of OT which increased team members' understanding, and led to more appropriate referrals and acceptance of the new focus of our work. These are discussed below.

At the time of the re-evaluation of the OT service, an OT managed us and was supportive of the change in direction. She recognised the core skills of OT and read the literature that supported the new interventions. She encouraged us to apply theories to practice and evaluate the results. This was invaluable. A sense of a team spirit among the OTs also meant that we were supported through good and difficult times, though not everyone was in agreement initially. Groups of three or four met on a monthly basis for peer supervision that focused solely on interventions we were doing with clients. This helped with solving any difficulties we were having, and also meant we learnt from each other's experiences. Such sharing of ideas developed our pool of resources. Literature on dementia care helped us to justify our focus on occupation, as did the literature on occupational science. Both were vital in enabling us to promote our role and explain to colleagues why we were doing activities such as baking, sewing, using music and gardening, etc. We were able to show that such activities were more than simply pleasurable, or something to keep a person quiet for a while. We demonstrated that such occupations are vital to a person's sense of well-being. At times people did not understand what our role was, while some who did were unappreciative of the complexity of analysing activities and adapting them. Colleagues, relatives, formal and informal carers all needed to recognise this, and the need for us to explain it clearly was crucial for any intervention to succeed and be continued by others.

Such a change in direction was a move away from the classic medically driven emphasis on diagnosing people and simply providing medication and care packages. The whole culture of our dementia care changed. We considered who people were, how they felt and what they did. Our measures of success depended not on the absence of problem behaviours, but on the presence of signs of well-being. We looked for self-expression, relaxation, the initiation of communication and a sense of belonging, etc. It did not happen overnight; our skills developed with practice and continue to develop as we continue to learn from those with dementia and their carers. The support of others was vital in all we did. Mostly, having a sense of the person with dementia, spending time finding out what motivated them and knowing something of their life story inspired us.

There are still times when, due to pressure of work, we are unable to focus on occupation as fully as we would like. However, we are immensely proud of the way we have refocused, as many other OTs describe the frustration of recognising occupational needs, but feel unable to change their work style. In many ways this indicates the future need for OT in dementia care. We have shared our journey with many people at study days and conferences, yet we need to share it more, as do others with similar journeys from which we can learn. We need to evaluate our interventions more rigorously and demonstrate the benefits of occupation for well-being. This will enable others to use such evaluation to justify why they need to address such needs. So far we have found the well-being profile devised by the Bradford Dementia Group (Bruce, 2000) helpful in evaluating the impact of our interventions. This is devised in such a way that it is easy for others to understand. Other measures, such as dementia care mapping and single system methodology, are excellent evaluation tools, and there are more waiting to be devised that will be invaluable. We need to generate the need to have them.

In conclusion, since addressing people's occupational needs, our job satisfaction has increased immensely. There has been a cultural change in the way we deliver care, and we feel that we have learnt so much more about dementia and the way it can affect people's lives. It has helped us really to meet people with dementia, rather than simply seeing the problems associated with dementia. There have been moments of intense sadness when recognising a person's losses, and times of sheer joy when we have been with someone engrossed in an activity. The rewards of positive feedback have come from the people we have worked with, their families and formal carers.

After the death of Moses, his son commented that the life story book that had been done with his father had not only been an enjoyable process for Moses, but had helped his son talk with him towards the end of his life, as they could chat about the photographs in it without needing Moses to remember details as they were written down. He felt it was now a beautiful reminder of the person Moses had been, which helped the family to remember him outside of the context of his dementia.

Our final thought is one of encouragement. If you are working with people with dementia, recognise and address their occupational needs. It will enhance their lives and those around them. Experience has taught us it can take a great deal of time before success is achieved. It may involve some trial and error before an activity is found that meets a person's occupational needs. It is clear, however, that when you find that activity and observe the enjoyment on the face of the person there is nothing better for the well-being of the person involved, or your own job satisfaction.

Appendix – Leisure Interest Checklist

Client's Name _____ DoB _____

OT _____ Date _____

	Have you ever had an interest in (please tick)	Details
1 Recreations Indoor games, eg chess, cards, scrabble, etc. Sports Art appreciation Countryside & wildlife eg birdwatching/walks Bingo/betting, eg lottery Horseracing Reading, eg books/magazines		
2 Hobbies Collecting, eg stamps Pets Gardening – indoor, outdoor DIY Crafts, eg painting, sewing, knitting, etc Cooking for pleasure Photography Swimming Dancing Fishing Playing/singing music Computers		

continued

Appendix – Leisure Interest Checklist (continued)

Client's Name _____ DoB _____

OT _____ Date _____

	Have you ever had an interest in (please tick)	Details
3 Holidays/outings Day trips Holidays Visits to stately homes Visits to historic buildings Cycling Driving Shopping		
4 Entertainments Television Radio Video/films Going to shows/theatre Cinema Listening to music Socialising Eating/drinking out Entertaining at home Social clubs		
5 Volunteering/ organisations Voluntary work Church activities Club/organisation Member/committee member		

continued

Appendix – Leisure Interest Checklist *(continued)*

| Client's Name _____ DoB _____ |
| OT _____ Date _____ |

	Have you ever had an interest in (please tick)	Details
6 Education Classes		
7 Employment		

CHAPTER 12

Changing A Culture:
The Westminster Project

Richard Mepham

'Just one more thing – It's been emotional'

Quotation from *Lock, Stock and Two Smoking Barrels,*
directed by Guy Ritchie.

In the UK we know a thing or two about heroic failure: there was Captain Scott's mission to the South Pole for one, the charge of the Light Brigade for two and the majority for our sportsmen and women for three. No other nation in the world displays such skill at snatching defeat from the jaws of victory. Yet perhaps there is something about all this in the national psyche that makes failure so difficult for us to swallow.

Failure is a thing of beauty. It gives us the opportunity to display humility and a philosophical outlook and that should be cherished (as anyone who has supported Ipswich Town Football Club for as long as I have will tell you!). But, most importantly, to deny failure is to deny learning and, in turn, to deny knowledge. No learning experience is possible without failure. Consider Captain Scott again. He embarked on a scientific expedition to the South Pole that contributed to the development of knowledge, and, ultimately, the establishment of a world-renowned polar research centre, while his opponent, Amundsen, took a load of dogs and a sled to race there. Where is Scott's failure in that?

Parents often have a deep desire to help their children avoid the mistakes they have made in their own lives. They can express this through being controlling, which can drive the child to establish an identity by making his own mistakes, generally spectacular ones.

The point is that, without the freedom to fail and learn by failure, we are all doomed to make some monumental mistake at a later date, because we just have not learnt anything. This is true in the areas of both project work and activity provision. If we do not try something, evaluate the impact, adjust the approach and try again, then we get nowhere, very fast.

It is important to consider the nature of failure briefly, as, from some angles, the Westminster Project that I am going to write about here could be seen as less than successful. In truth it has been an important learning curve for all concerned. The lessons from this project must not be lost and need to be valued in the right way. What is the Westminster Project (or rather what was it)? Well, on the surface it was a two-year project to improve activity provision in four care settings for older people in Westminster, financed by both health and social services funds. It was my job to lead the project from start to finish as project officer, and personally it almost became my Waterloo. It has been an endeavour that has taken me through some highs, lows and even some amusing moments along the way. It has also provided me with a good grounding in the finer points of project management.

At the best of times project work requires efficient cooperative working from numerous parties, and the Westminster Project was no exception. This chapter is an attempt to look back on the project, the progress and the resultant lessons, not just for the benefit of others trying to improve activities, but also for those trying to lead projects of any type.

Naturally all names have been changed to protect the guilty, the innocent and the embarrassed.

Let me first set the scene: as stated, the project was funded by the healthcare trust and social services. In previous years the area of activity provision in older people's care settings had been highlighted as requiring improvement. The National Association for Providers of Activities for Older People (NAPA) was invited to submit a proposal for a project aimed at improving provision and duly submitted a three-year project outline. The funding bodies were not keen on the initial proposal: it was too long and not specific enough to the requirements of Westminster's long-term care providers. NAPA amended the proposal and resubmitted a one-year project comprising action research in four long-term care settings for older people, leading to an in-depth report and recommendations for developing the activity cultures. This specification allowed for the possibility of a second year, with NAPA assisting and advising as the care settings implemented the recommendations made for their environment. This project proposal and the second year option were accepted by the funding body and preparations began. This is where I enter the story.

In July 2000 I was appointed to the post of Project Officer. NAPA was looking for someone with a degree education, good interpersonal skills, experience in services for older people and, I suspect with hindsight, something of a thick skin. I fitted the bill: psychology background, day centre and continuing care ward experience – and a skinhead haircut. Little did I know at the time just exactly what it was that I had let myself in for.

As you would expect, I was not totally alone in my endeavours. Supervision was provided by NAPA's Director of Training, while other NAPA representatives were available for support and inspiration where required. A steering committee was assembled from management representatives of each project venue, a NAPA representative, myself and our social services link person. Social services provided Jane, a link representative from their older adults team, whose role was to empower me with local knowledge, make the necessary introductions at each venue and oversee the steering committee.

The care settings involved in the project embraced some diversity. Essex House was a privately owned large care setting with over 100 beds. It contained residential and nursing units for older people experiencing both mental and physical frailty. Sussex House and Kent House were both social services residential settings each offering approximately 45 places, while Surrey House was the only mental health trust venue and offered 20 places on a continuing care basis. Each venue volunteered to be involved in the project, although I suspect a degree of persuasion may have been employed in certain cases. So, with the formalities of introductions completed, the real work began. At this point it is probably most appropriate to give a brief overview of progress at each venue over the two years.

Kent House

Kent House was a cheery place to work and a nice environment to run a project of this nature. Staff, management and residents all got along very well and seemed to have each other's interests at heart. This was reflected in warm relations between staff and residents, and the fact that turnover among care staff appeared low.

Kent House had no experience of employing an activity coordinator, although funding had been approved and the search for a suitable candidate was about to begin. The vacuum in activity provision had been filled by a member of management who instructed care staff to lead on group activities for residents for one hour each afternoon. This manager passed around equipment and made activity suggestions to staff at the appropriate time each day.

Year one went smoothly enough and the research proposed a number of recommendations. For example, the care staff team was required to clean residents' rooms each morning, leaving little time for occupational engagement with residents. Indeed, on my first day of participant observation, I volunteered to vacuum the rooms on one unit, a decision I regretted an hour and a half and several buckets of sweat later. One of the resulting report recommendations, therefore, was for the domestic work undertaken by care staff to be stopped or vastly reduced to allow one-to-one time with residents and develop activity use outside the allocated hour each afternoon. A further report recommendation stated that activity notes should be kept and reviewed, and that residents be given a voice in planning the group and one-to-one activities they engage in. The home manager accepted all recommendations, but warned that domestic work arrangements were enshrined within contracts and business plans. The reallocation of domestic tasks was unlikely to be swift.

Year two began with a major hitch. It was expected that an activity coordinator would be in post before work to implement recommendations began. Unfortunately, this was not the case, and attempts to appoint an activity coordinator proved fruitless. Coupled with this, the member of management who had taken a lead in activities left, and care staff were too tied up with vacuuming rooms to get involved. Without a doubt, the situation appeared challenging no matter which way I looked at it.

Fortunately after I had spent a little time floundering (one resident accused me of being a police officer during a session in which unaccompanied by a member of staff, I had tried to ask her about activities she liked), another member of the management team offered to act as our link person and implement recommendations as far as he could. This manager was named Len. His involvement was voluntary and he seemed to take a great interest in the work and approach.

Len did the best he could with the time available, but, as ever at Kent House, the problems were time and resources. Together we gave residents a voice in activity planning by completing detailed assessments. We introduced staff to life history work, therapeutic planning in personal care and activities of daily living, and promoted note keeping and reviews in activity planning. The problem all along was that we could only promote ideas and show how staff could put them into action. The staff had no spare time to do any of it and neither did Len.

Despite this, I was able to see something that was perhaps more important: a shift in attitude. The home manager was very clear about the direction and use of activity that Kent House needed to employ. 'It's not about having a bus sitting out there to take a group out on a trip, it's about doing something with someone that actually means something to them. Doesn't matter what it is', she told me towards the end of the work. These were principles she had applied in her search for an appropriate candidate for the activity coordinator job, which was probably why no one had been found. Then, as if by some celestial providence and with all the comic timing of a broken alarm clock, such a candidate was appointed. This occurred just in time for the incoming staff member to wave me goodbye as the project ended. C'est la vie.

All in all, I believe that the project at Kent House was a success. Progress was made in difficult circumstances and with few resources. The place was left primed and raring to go with a better resource base, the right direction and all the tools to go a long way up the road towards good practice in activity provision. I left with my head held high and my reputation largely intact.

Essex House

Essex House was a new establishment. It was large and rather impersonal. It comprised six units, each with a locked door policy, promoting little contact between the residents or staff of different units. Staff that did switch between units found that the autonomous nature of each, and the different resident groups, almost gave the feeling that you had walked into another home entirely. The only thing negating this impression was the rather regimented, clinical décor throughout the whole establishment.

During the first year I worked as part of the team on two separate units and also spent some time with the activity staff. There was an activity staff team of three, covering the entire resident group from their own separate office. The majority of the rest of year one was spent pursuing the elusive home manager and deputy. These two appeared to have something of the Scarlet Pimpernel about them whenever I was in the building.

The key recommendation of the first year report, which both summarised year one and set the tone for year two, concerned cooperation. Activity staff complained bitterly about the lack of support they received from care and nursing staff. They reported on what they felt was a stressful job, sometimes reducing them to tears and made worse by an absence of cooperation from the wider staff team. This was all quite emotional and I felt quite moved. A recommendation was produced to suggest methods of improving cooperation, either by basing activity staff on units, requiring activity and care staff to plan and review activities together, or by interviewing care staff about what they could do to support activities, and encouraging them to engage in activity provision. Cooperation appeared the key theme and recommendation from year one. As it turned out, this was a little misleading and I could have focused my attention in other more profitable areas.

Year two commenced and continued for a good while in a frustrating manner. After initially accepting all recommendations in the presence of their newly appointed home manager (who replaced both the previous elusive home manager and her deputy), NAPA's Director of Training and Jane (our link from social services), two of the three activity staff had difficulty responding to the project and effecting the changes in practice required to implement recommendations. While not actually refusing any measure, they would tell me it had already been done, it would not work, or they could not see the point. If I left tasks for them, something more important always seemed to arise and prevent them from completing the work.

I began to feel even more concerned when I was asked to vet residents' artwork that was to be displayed to relatives during an activities event. It was suggested that I should remove all the 'age inappropriate' pictures likely to offend relatives. 'That's nursery school stuff,' one staff member remarked to a member of activity staff on seeing a model of an angel produced in the run-up to Christmas. I raised an eyebrow.

There seemed to be a general feeling among the wider staff team and observers that activity staff understood their roles as geared towards entertainment and producing tangible end products, rather than as purely therapeutic. Observation on my part revealed that large impersonal art groups had become the norm, with residents being urged away from their breakfasts still clutching newspapers and wearing confused expressions, as they were thrust into groups to colour in a tree, first thing in the morning. Challenging this, I asked to see an effort to work with residents individually and assess their use of activity. 'We can't do that. We've only just got these people into a routine', came the reply. I was puzzled, as I felt that getting people into a routine was not the function of activity staff, rather it should be the reverse. In the midst of this, I made full use of my supervision in order to retain direction.

Subsequent developments were equally disappointing. A couple of months later, having completed individual assessments for each resident with the activity staff, I left them for a couple of weeks to develop the assessment information. On my return, I found two activity staff responding to a physiotherapist who was reporting that a resident had expressed feelings of isolation to her, 'These people don't know what they are talking about, you can't trust what they say'. Strangely, I felt more hurt that activity staff could refer to their residents as 'these people', than that they believed the utterances of their residents were invalid. I was also puzzled that they would discourage other professions from sharing information, given that they had declared a lack of cooperation as being the greatest difficulty they experienced in their roles. I challenged both their perception of how confused residents communicate, and also their interactions with other staff members in the team. 'We don't need anyone coming round here telling us how to do our jobs' one of the activity staff told me, and I took this to be a thinly veiled threat. I felt it best to withdraw and consider the situation before any further damage to the working relationship occurred.

After taking supervision and discussing the situation with the home manager, I withdrew from Essex House. However, this was where Essex House began to make progress. The home manager spoke to each of the three activity staff and asked them to continue the work I had set, but under her supervision. While making great efforts initially, two of the team began to find providing a flexible, individual approach to activity provision very demanding. Shortly, both these staff members left Essex House, but not before destroying the individual assessments we had completed for 70 residents and sending the third activity coordinator 'to Coventry' for cooperating with the new programme.

The remaining member of the activity team was promoted and implemented a good deal of the directions to activity provision that we had discussed. A new team was built around her that had no preconceived ideas about the work. One unit even relished the chance to engage in the project without the support of activity staff, and instigated life history work and therapeutic planning in activities of daily living and personal care, using documents I had provided – so much for the entire care staff team being uncooperative in activities.

So at Essex House the phoenix rose from the ashes. What could have been an unmitigated disaster proved possibly the greatest success of the project. Much of the credit has to go to the home manager for intervening and not giving up on the project when I was at my lowest ebb. On reflection, it occurs to me now that the activity staff were right all along: the problem was all about cooperation, respect and support between the different professions within Essex House. But, as is so often the case, we all need a healthy dose of introspection and humility in order to solve any problem.

Surrey House

To a certain extent Surrey House did not need the input of this project as desperately as other project venues. There were obvious benefits for them in accommodating me, but activity provision was pretty well advanced in the first place. The entire staff team was well aware of the use of occupational engagement as a therapeutic tool and consistently employed it. There were a number of factors that made Surrey House a smooth ride for me. First, the management had in place a long-term activity training strategy that had benefited the entire staff team. They knew that use of activity was important and they knew that the project was important. Second, there was a history of employing qualified, experienced activity coordinators. Even though during the first year of the project the activity coordinator position was vacant, activity was still omnipresent at Surrey House. Third, being a healthcare environment, staff to resident ratios were better than in residential care, and so the staff team was under slightly less pressure.

The first year was unremarkable except for the fact that it had gone without a hitch (which probably was remarkable in comparison with other project venues). Recommendations were made regarding use of life history, therapeutic planning around activities of daily living and personal care and even individual goal planning, which I confidently predicted we could put into practice at Surrey House, such was the development of their system of activity provision.

It was toward the end of year one that Surrey House employed a new activity coordinator and they could not have found a better candidate. Jackie was skilled, experienced and qualified with a master's degree in recreation therapy from the USA. My cup ran over and joy was totally unrestrained! The possibilities were limitless. We breezed through implementing the recommendations with the support of the staff team. A new note-keeping system was set up to encourage nursing staff to record their activity work with residents, in-depth assessments of each resident quickly followed and we began to implement greater planning around activities of daily living. There was just one problem, albeit a delightful one: we were in a race against time, since Jackie was pregnant and poised to leave six months into year two. My cup had sprung a leak and was now rapidly emptying.

Prior to Jackie's departure, we worked with staff using life history documents, therapeutically planned activities of daily living for a sample of residents, and explored the feasibility of individual goal planning at Surrey House. All of this was a triumph and Jackie left on a high note to successfully bring a new life into world. I quietly sloped off to take some supervision and figure out where to go from here. The answer became clear very quickly. Staff covered for Jackie and continued to provide high quality therapeutic activity provision, as well as their normal high quality care. So where did I go from here? Well quite simply, and, as the saying goes, 'If it ain't broke don't fix it', I let them get on with it. Surrey House had the required documentation to implement all the recommendations and they had the know-how. What they did not have at that point was anyone with the time available to do it. Proper therapeutic activity provision is a full-time job that must be completed without distraction. I simply could not ask any member of the nursing team to take on this responsibility while simultaneously carrying out their own work.

I took a great deal of heart from working at Surrey House. In many ways Surrey House gave me the fuel to be able to face the challenges that my role threw up at other venues. It was a joy to be listened to, and to know that my work was regarded as important. It was disappointing not to be able quite to get that cherry on top of the cake, but it was a pleasure to have had some role in developing an exemplary activity culture.

Sussex House

Sussex House provided a challenge in every sense of the word. The research phase in year one was fine. Sussex House showed a strong tradition of activity provision and ran group sessions seven days per week. Recommendations from the first year report dealt primarily with clarifying the position of the activity provider (a lady named Josie who was actually employed as a care assistant) and developing activity provision supplementary to the existing group programme. Additionally, it was recommended that activity records be established and maintained to aid planning and reviewing activities for individual residents. All was well as the first year ended.

Between the end of the first year and the beginning of year two, Sussex House appointed a new manager called Ann. Ann accepted the project, sounding a few innocuous cautionary notes relating to resources, staff and the necessity to improve health and safety under her regime. With these comments noted, Ann left me to begin the work with Josie. To cut a long story short, fates and the number of different, conflicting roles held by Josie at Sussex House conspired to limit opportunity for our cooperative working initially. Each time I attended for a prearranged session, Josie (who also acted as health and safety officer) was unavailable, as she had urgent business to attend to with building contractors. On one occasion I waited patiently for two and a half hours, at the end of which time she was still unable to give me some attention. During the five weeks, illness and additional demands on her time meant that we were able to work together on only one occasion. This was through no fault of her own, but was not quite the flying start either of us had hoped for.

After the first month, Josie told me that since Ann had taken up post as manager few activity sessions had run, and none were likely for at least three months. This was principally due to Ann requiring Josie to attend to health and safety matters around the building, which she felt demanded urgent action. At this point I approached Ann and we discussed a way forward. Unfortunately, without access to a dedicated activity provider or some willing volunteer to take on that mantle, there was little I could offer. I raised this during supervision, and it was decided that I withdraw for a three-month period to allow health and safety issues to be addressed without the distraction of the project. It was also agreed that a meeting to revise expectations of what could be achieved during the remainder of the project term would be arranged by me.

Three months elapsed and, despite my being unable to arrange a meeting between my supervisor and the management at Sussex House (again fates and other commitments conspired to thwart my efforts), project work with Josie had commenced. Over four months late, we were now beginning work to implement recommendations. However, after only two sessions, similar problems began to re-present themselves: sessions had to be cancelled or restricted in duration so Josie could attend to health and safety issues.

In discussion with Ann I put forward my position, which was, in a nutshell, that progress in activity provision at Sussex House was unlikely, because they were unable to work with me at the present time. While being sympathetic, Ann was unrepentant; health and safety was simply priority and Josie was vital to this. Something had to give and it was the Westminster Project. The prevailing message was that, without sufficiently high health and safety standards, there was to be little or no therapeutic activity. Unfortunately, in the face of this notion, the point I was trying to make fell on deaf ears. My point was that a lack of activity provision in a residential care setting for older people is a health (if not a safety) issue. However, this impasse marked the end of the project at Sussex House. There was no anger, no animosity – just opposing perspectives. Activity provision lost.

The Lessons

The starting point of this chapter was to consider failure as a vital component of knowledge. While it is unfair to me and all other parties involved in the Westminster Project to classify it as a failure, it is fair to say that most of us expected to see a greater degree of development at our four care settings. However, this work was a unique endeavour that should be applauded, and was never likely to go according to any plan or expectations. It has been a learning experience.

Perhaps the Westminster Project's lasting legacy will be the acquisition of knowledge relevant to developing activity cultures in long-term care settings, rather than its contribution to the actual care settings involved. Reading through this chapter, I hope that key themes have presented themselves. I hope that readers have picked up on some of the issues they may face if attempting to develop activity provision in their own care setting. It may be useful here to revisit some of the key questions that must addressed in attempting to develop an activity culture.

Is there a good understanding of the health-related value of engagement through activity and a professional approach to its provision in the care setting?

Too often activity is seen as entertainment rather than therapy. This can lead to repetitive group programmes, a lack of individually tailored activities and very little therapeutic benefit to residents. Sussex House illustrates this well. There appeared to be little understanding of the necessity to provide activity. It was of low priority and the first aspect of service to be dropped when other issues arose. This lack of understanding was also evidenced by the fact that no activity records had ever been kept to use in planning and review of occupational engagement for individual residents. There was a limited understanding of what occupational engagement actually means, its vital nature, and little knowledge of how to go about providing it professionally.

Surrey House, on the other hand, had a good grasp of these issues. They understood the use of activity to enhance well-being and function. Their approach was well-documented and activity was planned with the needs of individual residents in mind. In fairness to Sussex House, it should be noted that Surrey House had made a significant ongoing investment in activity-related training for all staff members. However, the two approaches to activity provision could not have been further apart in terms of understanding, philosophy and approach.

Is there a clearly defined, long-term approach toward the development of activity provision that all the relevant parties fully understand and agree to? We learned that the planning for the Westminster Project was inadequate here; first, in that it was not long-term enough. The initial approach was to structure a three-year project. This was pared down to a one-year project and subsequently extended to two years. To a certain extent no one really knew how long it would eventually be. In my view, it would have been beneficial to all if the project had been planned, funded and administered over a fixed, three-year period that was not subject to alteration.

In terms of ensuring understanding and agreement among relevant parties, the project team and I should probably shoulder the responsibility. The approach altered dramatically between years one and two, from research to implementing recommendations. The impact of implementing these changes constituted nothing less than a shift in practice, attitudes and culture within each care setting. As a new type of project that was not being replicated from previous work, no one was really sure what the ramifications would be, and how they would be experienced at each venue. In fairness to ourselves, fully preparing any environment for such a leap into the unknown would have been next to impossible.

Are there sufficient resources available to develop activity provision and are they being utilised in the most effective way?

Kent House had considerable potential to improve activities because of their understanding of occupational engagement, but resource issues restricted development. They were insufficiently resourced in that they were unable to employ a dedicated activity provider to the staff team during the project. To compound this, although good resources were available in the form of a skilled care staff team, their role was inappropriate. Care staff had excellent key-working relations with their residents, yet they were required to spend each morning dusting, washing and vacuuming. These two resource issues undoubtedly restricted the benefits that Kent House could have taken from this project.

Is there a well coordinated approach to activity provision, comprising a shared responsibility across the staff team?

An effective system requires someone to take the lead in terms of planning, while providing activities with the support of a team. Surrey House employed an excellent, dedicated activity provider who was able to promote an advanced, individualised approach to activity provision for her residents, with the support of a well-trained staff team. Staff cooperated well, as they understood the value of occupational engagement because of the training they had received.

At Essex House it was a different story. The general staff team had little training and therefore little understanding of the value of activity (although care staff in one unit did demonstrate understanding and engage in the project under the direction of an astute team leader), while the activity team appeared isolated and unwilling, or unable, to do anything about it. A culture of blame had developed which had closed down effective communications. Coordination and cooperation are vital for the well-being of residents.

Do the relevant members of staff actually want the activity culture in question to develop and improve?

If the main players within a care setting do not want the activity culture to change, or do not see any room for improvement in activity provision, there is no chance of progress. Again, at Essex House two of the three activity staff saw no room for improvement in their practice. Indeed, they actually saw the recommendations and the work involved in implementing them as interfering with the approach they had settled on. Progress here was only made after these staff stepped aside and let others who did want change assume responsibility.

Is the manager informed, committed and enthusiastic about quality activity provision for residents?

If they are not, or do not understand the vital nature of occupation in relation to health, there should be some serious questions about the viability of implementing a programme of change. At Sussex House I found a manager who simply did not understand the importance of providing activities for her residents. She had suspended activity provision and required the dedicated activity provider to focus on her alternative role as health and safety representative. In this instance, I, or anyone else who entered the unit with an interest in activities, was swimming against a very strong tide. In short, there was no hope of improving activity provision. By contrast, after a difficult and unpromising start, Essex House achieved an incredible amount during the latter stages of year two, purely as a result of the manager understanding the necessity of the work and taking a strong lead.

This is the key: managers are all-important, and where their message is 'residents need therapeutic activity', or 'residents must have opportunity to satisfy their occupation needs', staff and the whole care setting will follow. Where their message is 'activity is not as important as X, Y and Z', little or no therapeutic activity will occur. In fact, you might as well rewind 25 years, turn on the television and just make sure that everyone looks clean and smells OK.

So, for me, the over all moral of the story is that if at first you don't succeed, try and try again. We are fully aware of the facts: without occupational stimulation people decline and generally begin to experience ill-being and ill-health. The approaches and tools to ensure that this does not happen are out there to be utilised; it is just a question of people picking them up and making the time to get on with it. Things might not go according to plan in the first instance, but that does not mean it is a disaster which should be forgotten about. It is a learning curve. The people you work with will benefit, and so will you in the end, if you just open yourself up to the possibility of failure and its two great friends, learning and triumph.

CHAPTER **13**

Collaborative Networking and Community Development: The Growing with Age Project

Sally Knocker

First lessons

I learnt to network very early on in my career. My brief as a community development worker was to work with older people on two large London housing estates to help foster neighbourliness and self-help for a group of senior citizens. These older people were becoming increasingly isolated and lacking in social opportunities in an area of London where expensive boutiques and large building societies had long since taken over from the butcher's and baker's shops.

As a 22-year-old novice, fresh out of university and full of energy and enthusiasm, I resolved to make contact with as many older people in the area as possible. I tried initially with a mail shot to the flats, introducing myself and the project, but received very little response. I decided therefore to take to the high street and the local gardens beside the church where many older residents seemed to spend their time. Gradually I was able to identify the key people in the area who could tell me a bit about the community in which I would be working. The supermarket and newsagent staff knew many of the pensioners by name. The postman told me about several older tenants who now rarely left their flats, and the estate manager, who seemed grumpy and unforthcoming at first, gradually opened up and started to chat. The women who did the flowers in the church had mothers who lived in the flats, and the gardener in the church gardens told me he was worried about an elderly couple where the wife looked exhausted and the husband seemed 'confused', dishevelled and seemed to 'shout a lot'. (I was later able to put this couple in touch with services which helped them.) By sitting in the garden on a summer afternoon, standing in the post office queue on a Thursday morning, or waiting at the bus stop, I started to meet the older people themselves. I found out more from them about the things that were concerning them and the improvements they would like to see. One man to whom I spoke told me how bored his wife (aged 75) had become, since retiring from being a secretary. I later recruited Gladys as an invaluable volunteer in my office and a key member of the social committee of older tenants, which I subsequently developed on the estate.

What is the relevance of this story to therapeutic activities you may ask? It is because 'community development' skills lie at the heart of the new culture of therapeutic activities. This induction period has stood me in good stead in all the subsequent jobs I have done. It is about having a curiosity and genuine interest to find out more about people and what 'makes them tick'; it is about making links with those who are the veins and arteries of that community, and finding new ways of bringing people together; it is about resourcefulness and friendliness and a good old-fashioned sense of neighbourliness, which the word 'community' conveys. The ability to network stems from an awareness of community that encourages an individual to look beyond their immediate doorstep to find other allies and supporters and to collaborate for mutual advantage.

The Dangers of Doing it All Yourself

One of the biggest challenges facing many activity organisers in care settings is making a decision about the extent to which they deliver activities themselves, and the extent to which they enlist the help of others. Many activity organisers are recruited because they are perceived as doers: they are often lively, practical people who are able to get on with running groups, organising outings and entertainers, etc. This kind of activity organiser has to learn to become more of an enabler than a doer if they are to bring in others to work with them. No wonder care staff and volunteers are less inclined to come forward to play a role in running social activities, if activity organisers appear so confident and competent that they are perceived as the only ones able to do the job well. The activity organiser who is able to take less of a centre-stage role and be more of a director, one who is able to nurture the talents and creativity of other 'actors', is likely, through delegation, to bring to the care home or day centre a much wider range of options. This activity organiser might be less in the limelight herself, but the end result might be many more hours in the week where a variety of things are happening and different people are involved.

The Growing with Age (GWA) Project

> Imagine a world where the local care home or sheltered housing scheme is the hub of community activity in an area, with doors open to a wealth of interesting experiences inside and outside the home – a place that people enjoy visiting, rather than dread that they might end up there.

This is the vision that has inspired the GWA project. The Growing with Age project, set up by the National Association for Providers of Activities for Older People (NAPA) in 2002, sought to explore the extent to which links with local communities could be harnessed to provide new outside interests and stimuli for elderly people living in care settings. There was recognition that there are many pressures on home managers, care staff and sheltered housing managers, and that they do not always have time to organise and run recreational activities. Through working closely with selected pilot sites across England, the project aims to find out how easy it is in reality to nurture links with a wider range of outside professionals and members of the local community who have distinctive contributions to make to the life of residents or tenants.

When defining what it is we mean by 'community', it can be helpful to do an informal 'map' of an area to get a sense of the kinds of individuals, groups, buildings and other resources that exist in the locality of a care home, day centre or sheltered scheme. This can sometimes reveal a surprising wealth of untapped possibilities, as Figure 13.1 on page 208 (based on a care home where I worked in central London) illustrates. As a result of doing this exercise, we started to make better use of what was on our doorstep. We had a number of enjoyable afternoons sitting on a bench opposite the entrance and exit to the local register office, for example, watching the wedding parties, reminiscing about wedding memories and commenting about the clothes, atmosphere, etc. The large children's playground proved a wonderful find. One woman in the very advanced stages of dementia, and who usually slept for much of the day, came to life with the colours and sounds of children playing, and started to clap her hands in delight as one little boy repeatedly came down the slide with great giggles. His mother brought the little boy over to the woman and they linked hands and smiles for several happy minutes. A contact at the local beauticians' college brought a number of young students to do facials and make-up demonstrations in the home, which gave pleasure both to those who had the direct experience and to those who watched. By attending the university's 'rag week', we recruited two very conscientious young male students: one acted as an escort to push a wheelchair on

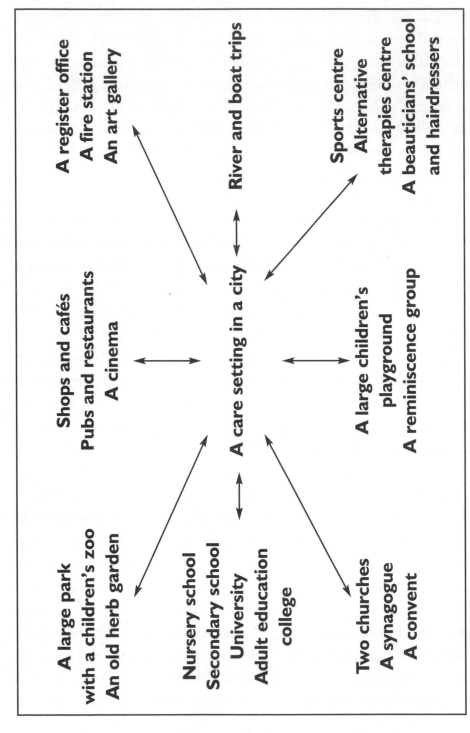

Figure 13.1 *Bridging the gap between the community and residential care*

occasional trips out, and the other played cribbage on a regular basis with a male resident who missed playing cards. These young men remained with us for the entire duration of their studies, over three years.

GWA has developed a list of potential contacts for care settings to explore, divided into three sections: 'Places to Go Out', 'Bringing the Outside In' and 'Students from Local Colleges'. *Care Settings in the Heart of the Community: Building a Local Resources Directory* (NAPA, 2002) offers activity organisers or other workers an opportunity to do an informal audit of their own area, with space to complete local contact details and other relevant information. The A-Z lists of ideas include over 140 possibilities to research, although of course much depends both on the type of locality and the interests and aspirations of older people in the care setting. It is hoped that one of the outcomes of GWA will be to produce a revised version of this directory for wider distribution.

Who is Living 'in the Community'?

A difficulty to overcome is in encouraging the wider public to perceive care homes as part of the community. The language we have used since the Community Care Act in 1990 has not assisted us here. We talk frequently about keeping people living 'in the community', which actually means staying in their own homes, so that by implication, when they have to move into a care home, they are somehow seen to be removed from that community. All the rhetoric has also contributed to the perception that this move is likely to be a last resort and something to be avoided if at all possible; a place to die rather than to live. When I asked a man what he felt about living in a residential home, he said, poignantly, 'It's like a hospice really; you get forgotten about here.'

The vision of care settings being in the heart of the local community requires a major shift in the way that many care homes and sheltered schemes currently operate. Net curtains need to come down, and busy managers need to look above the parapet of onerous paperwork and ever-increasing demands on their time and budgets to the sunnier horizons of creative partnerships with other organisations and individuals in the community who have something new to offer.

It is hoped that the specific mention of the importance of maintaining community links in the *Care Homes for Older People: National Minimum Standards* might put this issue more squarely on the agenda. Standard 13 states: 'Service users are able to have visitors at any time and links with the local community are developed and/or maintained in accordance with the service users' preference.' The crux of the issue is the extent to which care providers proactively investigate 'service user preferences' in this particular area, and whether 'community links' are interpreted more broadly and creatively than a visit from the chiropodist or a church service in the home every few months.

The project's initial research suggests that there are many potential friends and neighbours out there if we can find the time to reach out to them. Telephone calls to adult education colleges, leisure centres and museums reveal that there are often appointed officers with particular responsibility for outreach and support to older people. They are delighted to hear from a potential recipient for their services, and are open to exploring how they might be able to adapt what they offer to the needs of frailer older people.

Some of our pilot schemes are finding unexpected 'partners' in unusual places. One sheltered scheme has managed to recruit regular good quality and low cost entertainment through chatting to buskers in the local high street and enlisting their involvement. A care home has befriended a local ice-cream van that now calls weekly during the summer months and offers a special deal. Another care setting has developed a very productive partnership with a local college of English, and students are very keen to come and practise their English, offering companionship and conversation to older residents in return. This is an excellent example of the therapeutic relationship being one of mutuality and reciprocity.

Joining Forces towards a Common Goal

Neighbourliness and collaboration between care homes has also been successfully developed in the Darlington pilot site in two different ways. Many of the homes were suffering from a lack of accessible transport, so residents were very rarely able to get out of the home to go to the local shops or to visit areas of interest. Individual efforts by the homes to draw attention to the injustice that older residents in care settings were facing in terms of effectively being housebound fell on deaf ears. However, when the care homes teamed together and developed a collective voice, supported by a diligent local NAPA representative, the council relented and came up with a leased bus, which could be shared jointly between five homes. This now gives each home access to transport one day a week and on one weekend in five. Thus a shared problem has now resulted in an invaluable shared resource. The second way in which these homes have come together is to use this bus to visit each other so that informal tea parties are hosted in different homes, offering a welcome change of scene and a possible opportunity to meet new people. (It will be interesting to see if any residents decide to change home as a result of these visits.)

Potential Barriers to Community Involvement

It would be wrong to suggest that making links with the local community is always easy. Some communities are much more cohesive and open than others. Some care settings are located in streets in suburbs or remote rural areas far from any shops, parks, playgrounds, libraries or other facilities. Many residents of care homes find themselves living in an area with which they have little past connection, and their real 'home', in the sense of history and relationships with people, may well be several hours away.

There are also still many barriers to making care homes more open institutions, not least of which are important considerations such as the security and privacy of residents. The ideal of making care homes a resource for the community – for example running yoga classes which are open to older people living in the area, running an evening bar, or holding an art exhibition in the home to which outsiders would come – all bring serious implications, in terms of security. If we are really to treat a care home as a person's own home, then logically we cannot make it freely open to outside visitors. Yet by literally opening the doors to outside individuals and organisations, a care setting might start to free itself from its stagnant and depressing image. This delicate balance is something that the Growing with Age project seeks to explore further with its participating care homes and sheltered schemes.

Another area for consideration is the extent to which the need to organise (and pay for) checks on all volunteers through the Criminal Records Bureau might inhibit involving more outside visitors. Other blocks to making new links seem to relate partly to the increasing levels of frailty in older people living in care settings. It is difficult to assess whether this presents a real limitation to what people are in fact able to enjoy doing, or whether it represents more of an obstacle for staff members who cannot envisage that their residents would be able to benefit from these new contacts. In the example given above of the woman with advanced dementia visiting a playground, her care worker was astounded at her level of alertness and response to the experience.

However, this is not to underplay some of the challenges of inviting inexperienced 'outsiders' in to work with very physically or mentally frail people. In one care home, an adult education tutor who came in to do arts and crafts work left after two sessions. Initially the reason the tutor gave was that she felt these students (the older residents) were not going to be able to make progress, and so there was little point in continuing. It later emerged that the work had touched on some very real emotional issues for the tutor around her own losses, and these made it hard to be so close to frail older people.

We have as much to learn when these links with the community do not work out well as from the 'success stories'. Only then can we start to put in place the right kind of preparation to support appropriately individuals and organisations working with frailer older people or people with dementia for the first time.

Productive Partnerships

A great advantage of developing partnerships is that it opens up new possibilities for funding. Many funders consider approaches that come from a collaboration of organisations as particularly positive. This is presumably because they are aware that this funding bid is then likely to benefit from the investment of a good mix of skills and a cooperative effort, which will bring better results. By widening the horizons of creative activity for older people, there are infinite possibilities for potential partners in education, religious institutions, sports and leisure, horticulture and the arts, to name but a few. In order to develop these kinds of partnerships, we need to have a genuine willingness to be open to new ways of working and to being with people from different professional and personal backgrounds.

The Company We Choose

Many professionals in the health and social care field are used to working in splendid isolation. They might be surprised to discover that they could have colleagues who are ceramics artists, folk dancers or park rangers who might be able to bring something particularly enriching to a frail older person in a home. I remember having a conversation with one member of nursing staff in a home where we were talking about possible new visitors to invite in. I mentioned the idea of a visit from local firefighters or police officers, and she looked puzzled and said, 'Why would we want a visit from a fireman? What would they do?' This made me stop and think for a minute, until I remembered another recent discussion with a resident called Maggie who told me that she had a complaint to make about the home. This woman had a moderate level of dementia and seemed anxious to talk to me about her concerns. I asked her whether she would like to talk to the manager, and she said 'No, no, it's quite simple really'. She leant towards me to whisper quite intently in my ear at this point. 'There just aren't enough men in here!' All the residents at that time were women, as were nearly all the staff team. Maggie was a woman who had always thoroughly enjoyed men's company and was now understandably feeling their absence. The solution to Maggie's needs was not about what activity but more what kind of company she craved. If this was not available within the home, it made sense to make links in the community, which might well bring in more male visitors. For another resident, more contact with babies, young children or with animals might be more the kind of company the person was missing.

The View from the Window – Seeing Things from a Different Perspective

Recent years have seen many more arts projects in care settings: for example, musicians, artists, dancers and actors working with older people for a period of time. My own involvement in this kind of initiative has revealed that these sorts of artists bring a particularly fresh approach to their contact with older residents. Mutual involvement in the creative process seems to bring very special contact and pleasure, especially to those who have lost the ability to communicate as easily with words. Care workers can learn a great deal from working alongside workers who are less constrained by tasks and routines and more aware of here and now relationships and possibilities. One care worker who had been involved in an arts project said the one thing she had now learnt was to remember to look out of the window with residents. The artist had done a lot of work with residents and staff about the changing colours of the seasons, and the care worker now regularly sat with residents to look at the spring flowers, the autumn trees, the sun setting or the stormy clouds. She said this had brought many new benefits to her relationships with residents, partly because it made her stop and sit down for a time to take notice of the view from the window, but also because the sharing of beautiful or interesting things often felt quite magical and special for all those involved. This is an example of ways in which spiritual needs can be met at the most holistic level.

Listening to and Learning from Colleagues

We are all aware of the compartmentalisation and divisions that exist between different professions. Some of us would go so far as to say that each professional training gives you a separate language in which to communicate. This equips you to interact with your fellow professionals, but leaves you struggling with a dictionary when you encounter other professions with their own jargon. There are also situations where some practitioners are so precious about their particular role and contribution that they are unable to allow others in, lest they threaten that position in some way. Many professionals are at best suspicious of other professional groups, and at worst very negative and critical of the contribution they make. Stereotypes abound for almost all professions: the bossy and aloof nurse, the hippy or disorganised social worker, the 'nice' middle-class occupational therapist, the arrogant consultant doctor. We have probably all met at least one of these, as well as many others who do not fit the stereotype.

However, the last ten years have seen many more successes in multidisciplinary working, although we still have some way to go. Teams have been set up which include health and social services professionals, arts and complementary health therapists and care staff working in positive cooperation, with the shared aim of improving the quality of life of older people. These alliances work best where individual egos do not stand in the way of willingness to acknowledge the parameters of one's own expertise, and there is openness to learning from colleagues from very different fields.

One of the strengths of activity organisers is the diversity of their backgrounds and the resultant wide range of skills they bring with them. They are usually relatively free of any particular 'professional preciousness', as I call it. Some activity organisers come from a care work background, but I have met others who have come from assorted professions including a pub landlady, police officer, fashion designer, actor, supermarket manager and primary school teacher, to name but a few. While the need to raise the status of activity organisers as a distinct profession is extremely important, we need to be cautious not to make the academic requirements of any qualification so onerous as to lose potential applicants with great resources and personal attributes, but little formal academic background.

Large Organisations Nurturing Smaller Charities

The Growing with Age project is an example of a collaborative venture, since representatives from a range of large and small organisations conceived it as an idea. These organisations are Help the Aged, the National Institute of Continuing Adult Education (NIACE), the Open University and a sheltered housing group in the Gerontology Department of Sussex University. These partners recognised in NAPA a relatively new organisation with a very specific focus to support activity organisers. They gave NAPA practical support in putting forward a successful bid to the National Lottery Community Fund for the Growing with Age project. NAPA is responsible for managing the project, but the partners advise and monitor developments through participation in an advisory group. The bigger name partners will be particularly valuable to the project in its final stages. GWA will need their contacts, reputation and resources to conduct a much wider publicity campaign than NAPA can undertake on its own. This is a good example of where a large charity like Help the Aged can support and enable a smaller organisation to do a particularly creative and specialised piece of work, without taking it over.

Some larger organisations are more territorial and expansionist in approach, and small charities are more likely to sink than swim in this kind of climate, as competition for resources continues to be so tight. This will be regrettable, since much pioneering work stems from little specialist organisations representing the voice of a particular group and an important vision.

Last Lessons

This chapter has sought to emphasise how important it is to forge links and develop partnerships across many different fields of work and walks of life, in order to extend the opportunities for company, occupation and interest available to older people in care settings. Normal life includes small everyday opportunities to engage with and enjoy a variety of people, places and experiences. It is clear that it is not possible for the best of care staff teams to provide this range without support. Like all good partnerships, work needs to be done on both sides to help them succeed. Activity organisers need guidance and training to develop their skills in reaching out to, and making the most of, local resources, and to make these links meaningful and sustainable. Community organisations and other facilities need to be reminded that older people living in care settings are indeed part of their community, and to learn about how they might offer more to this neglected group of local citizens. They also need to be made more aware of the possible contributions that older people can make to the community, so that the relationship is one of exchange and mutual advantage.

The Growing with Age project is an example of a number of exciting developments in the sector, in which care professionals are learning to forge alliances in other fields, so that older people can continue to feel involved, included and valued in the wider world.

CHAPTER 14

NAPA: Steering the Path from Entertainer to Reflective Practitioner

Simon Labbett

What NAPA Stands For

NAPA is the National Association for Providers of Activities for Older People. It is a registered charity and a company limited by guarantee, and it is the only national organisation dedicated to:

- promoting activity in elderly care settings;
- supporting the work of people working in care settings to provide stimulating, meaningful activity.

Throughout this book the value of meaningful activity and of having fun in the process has been made abundantly clear. But what of the people whose job it is to stimulate that activity and generate that fun? If the value of activity is becoming so widely recognised, why is it that the role of the activity provider continues to be a struggle against poor working conditions, lack of understanding from colleagues and few prospects for personal development?

NAPA exists to represent the interests of these people. Without well-trained, well-motivated staff to deliver activities, care organisations will always be under-providing for those in their care. What NAPA stands for is thus simply stated. How it sets out to achieve this will be dealt with later. First, however, it would be illuminating to see why NAPA came to into being in the first place.

The Origins of NAPA

When people start talking of 'meaningful activity', 'purposeful occupation', or even 'activity used therapeutically', they are using the language of the occupational therapist (OT). The concepts of therapeutic intervention and purposeful activity are what drive occupational therapy. Work with older, frail people has to be one of the principal areas of engagement for the OT profession. Yet it is apparent that the profession has critically failed to address a pressing need in the residential and nursing home sector.

The last 15 to 20 years have seen the nature and abilities of the typical care home resident change markedly. The pressing need has been for skilled staff in these homes to engage with the increasingly frail, disabled and dependent clients who were living there. The role of such staff clearly required the individual to possess three basic areas of aptitude:

- the ability to be creative, spontaneous, resourceful and good at engaging with people at an appropriate level;
- the ability to be reflective and to have insight into how older people react to, and function within, a care setting;
- to understand what motivates people and how to plan activities thoughtfully to achieve certain aims.

I suspect that home owners were (and still are) generally more inclined to appreciate the value of the first area of aptitude. This is hardly surprising. An individual with a little flair and 'people skills' can generate signs of activity fairly quickly, particularly with the more motivated residents, and thus create a home with a sheen of life and colour. This is what visitors to the home see and comment on, and should give the home owner the sense that their financial investment in activity provision has been well spent. In contrast, one suspects that some home owners still see activity organisers as entertainers, and are far less persuaded of the need for such staff to plan activities as an integral part of the care package.

Yet it is the view of some in the occupational therapy profession that it was this same creative and inventive area of aptitude that the occupational therapy profession neglected. In an article in the *British Journal of Occupational Therapy* in 2001, Tessa Perrin contends that OTs turned their back on their original raison d'etre which was rooted in the creative processes of arts and crafts provision, and consequently neglected to focus on the relationship between creativity and health.

As Perrin points out, by the 1990s the 'occupational and creative' needs of clients in residential homes were starting to be addressed, but only rarely, by OTs. The impetus was coming from diverse disciplines such as nursing, psychology and even business. Furthermore, the people who delivered the activities were often not professionals at all, but unqualified, untrained members of the care team or private business practitioners.

The activity business was growing fast. However, it was growing in a haphazard way and with very little theoretical underpinning. It is inevitable that with such rapid growth some questionable practice would occur, even where it was done with the best of intentions, and that this practice was being passed on as acceptable. In short, the second group of skills was being neglected.

A fledgling profession was being born. By the middle of the 1990s a need clearly existed for an organisation that could attempt to bring together such disparate practice and map a future. Such an organisation needed to:

- offer means of practical support to activity providers and homes;
- voice the needs and concerns of the activity provider;
- research and share good practice;
- set bench marks for good practice;
- lobby for recognition of the value of activities and providers of activities.

It was a tall order that required vision. It found that vision in two non-UK nationals. The impetus to found NAPA came from Mariana Boneo, who was trained and worked as a music therapist, and John Reilly, who had trained and worked as a psychotherapist, but at that time was working as an activities organiser in London. Mariana had been part of a special interest group at Bradford University for those providing activities in care settings for older people. This group ran for a limited period only, but by the time of its closure Mariana had caught the vision and returned to London to set up the formal organisation that in due course came to be known as NAPA.

The initial group of individuals who worked with Mariana and John includes many names who are still very actively involved with NAPA's work. But it was not just a question of individuals; it was also the organisations and professions that they represented. NAPA needed (and received) representation from organisations and professional bodies that had a stake in the overall state of UK care provision. Voices from the voluntary sector included Age Concern, Help the Aged, Counsel and Care, Alzheimer's Society, Residents' and Relatives' Association, Royal National Institute for the Blind, and from professions such as occupational therapy, nursing, gerontology, music and drama therapy. It is almost certain that this breadth of professional experience and organisational perspective, coupled with the energy of the individuals in question, has allowed NAPA to gain credibility swiftly, and has contributed to the sense of continuity in the organisation's growth.

The organisation's growth has, indeed, been swift. Mariana and John founded NAPA in 1997, by which time Sharing Days were well established. Sharing Days bring together activity providers to discuss issues of common concern and, since the days are practical in nature, to try out ideas and techniques useful in the workplace. The first members' newsletter was produced in 1997. Sharing Days and the newsletter rapidly became the two principle services provided for NAPA members. By the end of 1998 NAPA achieved charity status, held its first conference to draw attention to the issues, and launched its first regional group.

Defining the Profession

However, probably the biggest factor in taking the organisation's major ideas forward was the appointment of an experienced occupational therapist as Director of Training in 1999. This was the opportunity needed to offer more than support; this was the chance to set standards.

In 2001 NAPA published the document *Therapeutic Activities and Older People in Care Settings – A Guide to Good Practice*. It was written by the Director of Training, and was one product of an innovative project that NAPA undertook with (and was funded by) the City of Westminster to research how activities are provided in four differing settings within the authority.

The *Guide to Good Practice* is a definitive statement of what NAPA considers should be best practice in the provision of activities in care settings. As the author makes plain, the beliefs and standards that are stated in the guide pre-existed NAPA, but NAPA has brought to bear the greatest weight of knowledge in this field in the UK and has been responsible for uniting these beliefs, documenting them and putting them into practice. Most significantly for the fledgling profession, it is this document that sets out NAPA's view on the way activity provision should be resourced.

Two roles are clearly identified and differentiated: the activity therapist or coordinator and the activity organiser or provider. Leaving aside the sometimes thorny issue of job titles, NAPA is clearly stating that activities should be delivered according to a programme of individual goal planning, and that the person who coordinates this should therefore be fully integrated within the care planning process of a residential setting. Logic therefore dictates that the activity therapist/coordinator should have the same status and pay as junior management.

The role of activity therapist/coordinator clearly requires that the individual possess a level of insight into the way activities are delivered, monitored and assessed which would not be demanded of a 'standard' activity organiser, whose role focuses more on pure delivery. Such insight and management needs a greater degree of training than has hitherto been the case. Within the field of training lies another of NAPA's major achievements: the development of nationally recognised accredited training for the activity coordinator.

The City & Guilds Progression Award 6977 – Certificate in Providing Therapeutic Activities for Older People – was developed by NAPA and gained accreditation in the summer of 2002. It has an notional equivalence to NVQ Level 3, and, as such, is clearly targeted at the more experienced activity provider (as outlined in the Good Practice Guide). The five units are: human ageing in health and illness; delivering therapeutic activities; the effective use of resources; interpersonal communication; activities; and a therapeutic resource. Of course it remains to be seen what the take-up will be for this course. The awarding body takes responsibility for marketing such courses, but it would be naive to think that NAPA could sit back and wait for it to be taken up in droves. Home managers will need to be convinced that it is a wise use of resources. Clearly we hope that they are convinced, but training budgets are vulnerable when money is tight.

Of course NAPA recognises that the vast majority of activity sessions will continue to be provided by designated activity providers or members of the care team who have other duties to perform. NAPA believes that the best way to help them in their practice is through Sharing Days, training days and information sharing via the newsletter and website. Wherever appropriate, Sharing Days consistently aim to provide a theoretical basis to support the subjects that are covered. Our belief is that not only does this provide a firmer underpinning to an activity organiser's way of working, but it also gives them a rationale for the activity to pass on to a line manager, inspector or relative who might be of the sceptical persuasion.

Resourcing NAPA

It should be clear from the foregoing that NAPA has benefited from a number of factors which, when combined, create fertile organisational growth. There has been the timeliness of the issues (recognised and reinforced by government legislation), a strong collective desire to preach a message, a reassuring number of influential organisations and individuals who have responded to that message, and, above all, a unique selling point. This is that it is the only organisation working exclusively in this area. Regrettably, timeliness, energy and respect are not in themselves a guarantee of longevity. Financial resources have no small part to play.

NAPA is largely run as well as managed by its trustees – a situation familiar to some smaller charities, but one ill-befitting a national organisation. Furthermore, like a very large number of other small and medium-sized charities, the organisation faces enormous problems in securing funding for core costs. The way ahead lies with specific project funding (as opposed to funding which only finances core costs). Here NAPA has become increasingly successful: the sense that funding success breeds further funding success is pleasing once finance has come in, but hardly a helpful strategy when you are just starting out.

The Department of Health is shortly to fund key information and advice work, and we are currently in the latter stages of a three-year project funded by the Commmunity Fund. This project, 'Growing With Age', is all about researching good practice and sharing it (see Chapter 13). Growing With Age has set out to map the links that care homes and sheltered housing networks are making with the community, both in terms of the home reaching out and the community coming in. Apart from the stability that this project has brought to NAPA, perhaps the most heartening thing about it has been the attitude of NAPA's partners in the bid towards us. They not only valued the work that the project proposed to undertake and felt sure we were best placed to undertake it, but also saw it as a way of gaining recognition for NAPA generally, and enabling us to raise our profile. This attitude rather runs counter to the notion that larger organisations will tend to manipulate or devour smaller ones. I suspect that, to a greater or lesser extent, the way forward for many smaller charities will be to create mutually beneficial working arrangements with the larger players in their particular broad field.

The Future

In this chapter we have been looking at the development of a fledgling profession which has grown in tandem with an organisation whose remit is to work on behalf of that profession. Few would dispute that NAPA has been hugely influential in fostering the growth of that profession, particularly when viewed in relation to its meagre resources, but does this mean its work has been done? Where does NAPA go now?

The stark reality is that daily life in care can still be numbingly boring and soul destroying. For every beacon of good practice, or even of goodwill, there are an equal number of people who do not see activity and occupation as an essential part of caring. I feel that NAPA's twin objectives of campaigning and supporting are still as valid as ever.

Lobbying for a Greater Role for Activities

While the Care Standards Act and the National Minimum Standards do draw attention to activities, the crucial question relates to how the new Commission for Social Care Inspection will interpret the Act in relation to this area. For the individual home being inspected, what constitutes a failure in this area? If they have 'failed', what is deemed a sufficient improvement and what evidence will be required? Such judgements imply a bottom line of acceptability. It is doubtful that either the resident or their family would find that bottom line acceptable. More pertinently, what is the Commission's knowledge and attitude to the subject, and what sort of importance will they place on it in the wider scheme of things? It seems clear that if person-centred activity provision is enshrined in law (albeit rather vaguely), then NAPA's priority must be to work with the body whose responsibility it is to enforce that law. There are many bodies (not least the care providers) waiting to see what line the Commission will take in all areas of their remit. Fortunately, it is evident that NAPA is not alone in its concern for quality of life issues. One hopes that these other organisations will look to us for expert guidance, while using their greater organisational muscle to influence change.

There is a strong business case to be put for care home owners spending money on resources that create a vibrant and dynamic home environment. The future purchasers of care are of a different breed, and, the expectations of today's 60- and 70-year-olds will demand something more in keeping with their present experiences. One suspects and hopes that the days of the care home existing in splendid isolation in the community are numbered. In this context, NAPA's ongoing work, looking at the ways in which the care home can redefine its role in the community, deserves attention. NAPA should exist to assist home owners who are new to activity provision to plan their resources sensibly and to set realistic expectations for what can be achieved.

Professional Standards

In the absence of any leadership from other sources, NAPA has attempted to define the benchmarks of what an activity provider does. Yet it should be recognised that NVQ-equivalent accreditation is pitched at a level that will suit experienced activity providers, but will not suit the majority. The majority of activity providers, or care staff providing activities, are young and relatively inexperienced and will require different support (see Chapter 9). NAPA must consider its response to this carefully, and not just leap into creating yet another NVQ Level 2 (or equivalent) qualification.

Then there is the question of whose preserve it is to monitor the new profession and ensure that its aims are allied to other professionals working in the same field of healthcare. This begs a further question: at what level of engagement with activity provision does the practitioner become part of a profession? Certainly, the standards set by the City & Guilds award require a level of awareness and style of approach that surely dictate recognition by a professional body. As has been stated earlier in this chapter, NAPA has always had strong links with professional occupational therapists and the OT profession's ethos has underpinned much of our approach. There are signs that closer working with the College of Occupational Therapists may develop, which must be a positive step. However, we are not really talking about occupational therapists; we are talking about activity therapists (to chose the more controversial name, in order to highlight the difference). In the United States and Australia the occupational therapy profession and the body of fledgling activity professionals failed to reach an understanding. As a consequence, a whole new profession was born – the diversional or recreational therapist. I feel that NAPA would view such a move here as unnecessary and a failure on the part of those concerned to reach an understanding. What of those providers of activities, mentioned earlier, who are trained to operate at a lower level? Who will look after their interests if they are not part of a professional body?

One might expect the spokesman of any organisation to argue that its existence is entirely justified, and that is indeed the conclusion to which I have come. However, the voluntary sector is littered with organisations that have similar objectives to each other and target identical and limited sources of funding. The sector is also littered with organisations that fail. Therefore NAPA, like any other charity, needs to examine whether it is still achieving what it set out to do, to look at who is doing allied work, and to consider how it cooperates with other organisations without compromising its identity. Organisationally NAPA is in its infancy, but it speaks with a mature voice. It is still a necessary voice, but also a fragile one. For NAPA's trustees, the coming years will require the same energy and foresight to ensure the organisation's survival as it took to get it off the ground.

References

Allen C, 1985, *Occupational Therapy for Psychiatric Diseases: Measurement and Management of Cognitive Disabilities*, Little Browne, Boston.

Anderson TD, 1997, *Transforming Leadership: Building the Leadership Organization*, Blackhall, Dublin.

Archibald C, 1990, *Activities*, Dementia Services Development Centre, Stirling.

Armstrong-Esther C, Browne K & McAfee J, 1994, 'Elderly Patients: Still Clean and Sitting Quietly', *Journal of Advanced Nursing* 19, pp264–71.

Bandler R & Grinder J, 1979, *Patterns of Hypnotic Techniques of Milton H. Erickson*, Meta Publications, California.

Barker EM & Davidson D, 1998, 'Power and Control', McCormack B (ed), *Negotiating Partnerships with Older People*, Ashgate, Aldershot.

Best C, 1998, 'Caring for the Individual', *Elderly Care* 10(5), pp20–4.

Boyce T, 2001, 'Coping with the Stress of Caring', Cohen D & Eisdorfer C (eds), *The Loss of Self*, Revised edn, Norton, New York.

Bradburn N, 1969, *The Structure of Psychological Well-being*, Aldine, Chicago.

Bruce E, 2000, 'Looking After Wellbeing: a Tool for Evaluation', *Journal of Dementia Care* 8(6), pp25–7.

Campbell J, 1998, 'Living with Hope', *Candis*, October, pp40–4.

Centre for Policy on Ageing (CPA), 1996, *A Better Home Life: A Code of Good Practice for Residential and Nursing Home Care,* CPA, London.

Chapman A & Illesy J, 1992, *Paying the Price,* Dementia Services Development Centre, University of Stirling.

Chaudhary H, 2002, 'Place-biosketch as a Tool in Caring for Residents with Dementia', *Alzheimer's Care Quarterly* 3(1), pp42–5.

Clough R, 1999, 'The Abuse of Older People in Institutional Settings – the Role of Management and Regulation', Stanley M, Manthorpe J & Penhale B (eds), *Institutional Abuse: Perspectives Across the Life Course*, Routledge, London.

Coleman P, Ivani-Chalin C & Robinson M, 1993, 'Self Esteem and its Sources: Stability and Change in Later Life', *Ageing and Society* 13(2), pp171–92.

College of Occupational Therapists, 2002, *From Interface to Integration,* College of Occupational Therapists, London.

Cooper J, 2002, 'The Human Rights Act and Care Homes', *Nursing and Residential Care* 4(6), pp 286–8.

Covey SR, 2000, *Principled Centered Leadership*, Simon & Schuster, London.

Department of Health, 1998/2001, *Modernising Health and Social Services and All Our Futures: The Report of the Better Government for Older People*, Department of Health, London.

Department of Health, 2000, *Care Standards Act*, HMSO, London.

Department of Health, 2001, *Building Capacity and Partnership in Care*, Department of Health, London.

Department of Health, 2001, *Care Homes for Older People: National Minimum Standards*, HMSO, London.

Department of Health, 2001, *National Service Framework for Older People*, Department of Health, London.

Eales J, Keating N & Damsma A, 2001, 'Seniors' Experiences of Client-centred Residential Care', *Ageing & Society* 21, pp279–96.

Economic and Social Research Council (ESRC), 2001/2, 'GO: Growing Older Programme/Extending Quality of Life', *ESRC Newsletter,* 2 & 3.

Ely M, Meller D, Brayne C & Opit L, 1996, *The Cognitive Disability Planning Model*, University of Cambridge, Department of Community Medicine, Cambridge, cited in Kitwood T (1997), *Dementia Reconsidered: The Person Comes First*, Open University Press, Buckingham, p57.

Glass T, Mendes de Leon C et al, 1999, 'Population Based Study of Social and Productive Activities as Predictors of Survival among Elderly Americans', *British Medical Journal* 319, pp478–83.

Goldsmith M, 1996, *Hearing the Voice of People with Dementia: Opportunities and Obstacles*, Jessica Kingsley, London.

Gower, 1998, *Gower Handbook of Management*, 4th edn, Gower, Aldershot.

Henwood M, 2002, *Future Imperfect? Report of the King's Fund Care and Support Inquiry*, King's Fund, London.

Hird, Dame Thora, 2002, *The Sunday Times Magazine*, 6 January.

Holden C, 2002, 'British Government Policy and the Concentration of Ownership in Long-term Care Provision', *Ageing and Society* 22, pp79–94.

Innes A and Surr C, 2001, 'Measuring the Wellbeing of People with Dementia Living in Formal Care Settings; the Use of Dementia Care Mapping', *Ageing and Mental Health* 5(3), pp258–68.

Johnson M, 1994, 'Biographical Approaches to Health and Wellbeing', *Reminiscence* 9, pp3–4.

Jones M, 2000, *Gentlecare*, Haneley and Marks, Toronto.

Kelly M, 2002, 'A Health Promotion Strategy to Introduce Exercise Opportunities', *Nursing and Residential Care* 4, pp260–3.

Kitwood T, 1995, 'Cultures of care: Tradition and change', Kitwood T & Benson S (eds), *The New Culture of Dementia Care*, Hawker, London.

Kitwood T, 1997, *Dementia Reconsidered: the Person Comes First,* Open University Press, Buckingham.

Knocker S & Avila B, 2002, *Care Settings in the Heart of the Community: Building a Local Resources Directory,* NAPA, London.

REFERENCES

Laing W, 1998, *A Fair Price for Care? Disparities Between Market Rates for Nursing/Residential Care and What State Funding Agencies Will Pay,* York Publishing Services for Joseph Rowntree Foundation, York.

Lazarus RS, 1998, *Stress and Emotion: A New Synthesis,* Free Association Press Books, London.

Mullan P, 2000, *The Imaginary Time Bomb: Why an Ageing Population is not a Social Problem,* IB Tauris, London.

Nazarko L, 2002, *Nursing in Care Homes,* 2nd edn, Blackwell, Oxford.

Nolan M, Grant G & Nolan J, 1995, 'Busy Doing Nothing: Activity and Interaction Levels Amongst Differing Populations of Elderly Patients', *Journal of Advanced Nursing* 22, 528–38.

Pavlov IP, 1928, *Lectures on Conditioned Reflexes*: *1,* New York International Publishers, New York.

Perrin T, 1997, 'Occupational Need in Dementia Care: a Literature Review and Implications for Practice', *Health Care in Later Life* 2(3), pp166–76.

Perrin T, 2001, 'Don't Despise the Fluffy Bunny: a Reflection from Practice', *British Journal of Occupational Therapy* 64(3), pp129–34.

Perrin T, 2001, *Therapeutic Activities and Older People in Care Settings: a Guide to Good Practice*, NAPA, London (Speechmark, forthcoming).

Perrin T & May H, 2000, *Wellbeing in Dementia*: *An Occupational Approach for Therapists and Carers,* Churchill Livingstone, London.

Pietrukowicz ME & Johnson MMS, 1991, 'Using Life Histories to Individualize Nursing Home Staff Attitudes Towards Residents', *Gerontologist* 31(1), pp102–6.

Pool J, 2002, *The Pool Activity Level (PAL) Instrument for Occupational Profiling. A Practical Resource for Carers of People with Cognitive Impairment*, 2nd edn, Jessica Kingsley, London.

Richards M, 2001, *Long-term Care for Older People: Law and Financial Planning,* Jordan, Bristol.

Rogers C, 1959, 'Towards a Theory of Creativity', Anderson H (ed), *Creativity and its Cultivation,* Harper & Row, London.

Ross H, 1990, 'Lesson of Life', *Geriatric Nursing,* Nov/Dec, pp274–5.

Royal College of Nursing (RCN), 1992, *Nursing Homes: Nursing Values,* Royal College of Nursing, London.

Royal College of Physicians, Royal College of Nursing, British Geriatric Society, 2000, *The Health and Care of Older People in Care Homes: a Comprehensive Interdisciplinary Approach,* Royal College of Physicians, London.

Shenk D, 2002, *The Forgetting,* Harper Collins, London.

Soulsby J, 2000, *Fourth Age Learning Report,* Department for Education and Employment, London.

Sutherland S, 1999, *With Respect to Old Age: A Report by the Royal Commission on Long Term Care,* Executive Summary.

Telling M, 1998, *The Complete Guide to Long-term Care,* IFA Association, London.

Thompson N, 1999, *Stress Matters,* Pepar Publications, Birmingham.

University of Keele Centre for Occupational Studies, 1991, *Code of Practice for Staff Care in the Health and Social Services,* Local Government Training Board, Keele University, Keele.

Wilkinson H, 1998, 'Stress, Coping and Health in Families: Sense of Coherence and Resiliency', McCubbin HI, Thompson EA, Thompson AI & Fromer JE (eds), *Sense of Coherence and the Stress Illness,* Sage, London.

Index

A

activity
  coordinator v, xvii, 3, 19, 32, 36, 62,
    104–18, 140, 189, 190, 191, 194,
    195, 222, 223
  culture xiii, 4, 5, 9, 12, 45, 53, 116, 139,
    140, 196, 199, 202
    new culture xiii, xvii, xviii, 1–17, 49,
    52, 66, 69, 87, 109, 117, 135–46, 205
    old culture xvii, 1–17, 73, 86, 109, 141
  organiser xv, 6, 7, 8, 10, 38, 42, 44, 45,
    47, 53, 140, 141, 206, 221, 222, 223,
    224
  programme xvi, 4, 5, 45, 52, 63, 98,
    107, 127
  providers xv, xvi, xvii, xviii, 7, 8, 9, 13,
    52, 63, 73, 139, 140, 141, 142, 144,
    197, 198, 201, 202, 218, 221, 222,
    223, 226
  provision xii, xv, xvi, xvii, xviii, xix, 2, 3,
    4, 5, 6, 7, 12, 13, 17, 18, 26, 37, 38,
    40, 44, 52, 53, 55, 56, 59, 60, 64, 65,
    67, 71, 72, 86, 106, 107, 109, 114,
    119–34, 137, 139, 142, 146, 147–85,
    187, 188, 189, 191, 192, 194, 195,
    196, 197, 198, 199, 200, 201, 202,
    220, 222, 226, 227
    therapist xiii, 140, 222, 223
age-appropriateness 14
ageism 18, 22, 24, 25, 101
apprenticeship 141, 142, 144
assessment xvii, 23, 25, 51, 71, 73, 74, 78,
    79, 84, 86, 87, 98, 115, 144, 148,
    149, 154, 167, 168, 169, 171, 172,
    173, 174, 175, 190, 193, 194, 196,
    212, 223

B

books xv, 99, 128, 138, 153, 154, 156, 157

C

care plan 5, 52, 98, 120, 223
care process 4, 33
career structure 137, 139, 141
carers xiv, xv, 12, 20, 29, 38, 43, 45, 46,
    49, 50, 51, 61, 88, 89, 94, 95, 96, 97,
    102, 103, 144, 147, 149, 150, 157,

159, 160, 162, 163, 164, 166, 169, 171, 173, 174, 180, 181

City & Guilds 139, 141, 223, 227

cognitive impairment xi, 23, 31, 79, 80, 86, 136, 137

College of Occupational Therapists 139, 140, 227

Commission for Social Care Inspection 29, 225

community 19, 21, 27, 30, 32, 33, 35, 44, 53, 82, 94, 119, 124, 125, 126, 147–85, 205, 206, 207, 208, 209, 210, 211, 212, 214, 216, 217, 224, 225, 226

Community Care Act 21, 209

community development 204–17

craft 8, 10, 12, 43, 46, 107, 108, 130, 138, 139, 142, 143, 172, 212, 220

culture xiv, xvi, xvii, 1, 2, 10, 17, 18–38, 41, 42, 49, 52, 64, 65, 107, 110, 111, 114, 115, 116, 124, 137, 139, 141, 143, 145, 180, 186–201

D

day care 91, 100, 136, 137, 147, 148, 149, 150, 160, 163, 173

dementia xiii, xviii, 1, 10, 14, 21, 24, 25, 27, 31, 33, 34, 55, 56, 61, 64, 78, 81, 83, 86, 88, 89, 90, 91, 92, 93, 94, 95, 96, 97, 98, 102, 104, 105, 106, 113, 114, 123, 136, 137, 147, 148, 151, 153, 154, 161, 163, 165, 167, 168, 169, 171, 173, 174, 175, 176, 178, 179, 180, 181, 182, 207, 212, 213, 214

dementia care 1, 2, 59, 60, 109, 111, 147, 178, 180, 181

Dementia Care Mapping 86, 181

depression 2, 33, 76, 116, 148, 154, 155, 174, 212

disengagement 9, 11, 71, 72, 73, 87

diversional therapist 6, 19, 227

E

engagement xiii, 5, 6, 7, 9, 12, 13, 14, 32, 36, 40, 41, 44, 60, 65, 68, 71, 72, 73, 74, 75, 78, 79, 80, 83, 84, 85, 86, 92, 95, 104, 105, 107, 110, 113, 117, 135, 139, 142, 143, 168, 172, 174, 190, 192, 194, 195, 199, 201, 217, 219, 227

entertainment xvii, 4, 5, 72, 73, 86, 87, 140, 154, 172, 193, 199, 206, 210, 218, 220

equipment 53, 179, 189

F

fund-raising 13

funding 12, 13, 15, 16, 19, 24, 25, 32, 33, 73, 148, 165, 187, 188, 189, 200, 213, 222, 224, 227

G

Growing With Age xviii, 32, 36, 204–17, 224

H

home manager 38–70, 72, 93, 106, 190, 191, 192, 194

I

ideas xv, xvi, 3, 14, 42, 48, 50, 55, 57, 63, 67, 79, 88, 108, 115, 116, 117, 120, 122, 124, 126, 127, 134, 169, 172, 173, 174, 180, 191, 194, 209, 213, 216, 222

L

lifelong learning 18, 32, 36

long-term care xi, 18, 19, 20, 21, 22, 25, 26, 28, 35, 37, 39, 61, 72, 77, 87, 148, 188, 199

M

multidisciplinary 25, 33, 117, 215

music 12, 72, 73, 75, 76, 77, 81, 82, 85, 93, 108, 110, 128, 130, 153, 154, 157, 172, 174, 178, 180, 221

N

NAPA xviii, 19, 30, 32, 36, 139, 140, 141, 142, 145, 188, 192, 206, 209, 211, 216, 218–228

National Care Standards Commission 26, 28, 29

National Minimum Standards 29, 30, 34, 210, 225

National Service Framework 20, 29, 31, 32

negotiation 9, 11, 17, 62, 155, 163

nurses 39, 40, 41, 42, 43, 44, 46, 48, 49, 50, 51, 52, 55, 56, 64, 73, 99, 100, 105, 106, 148, 151, 164, 215

O

occupation xvi, xix, 11, 18, 19, 21, 26, 36, 54, 56, 57, 60, 64, 65, 68, 69, 83, 113, 116, 117, 118, 137, 138, 143, 146, 160, 168, 169, 174, 180, 181, 202, 217, 219, 225

occupational therapist 6, 36, 42, 43, 44, 46, 140, 168, 169, 172, 174, 177, 178, 179, 180, 215, 219, 220, 222

occupational therapy xii, xviii, xix, 6, 18, 19, 21, 25, 36, 42, 43, 45, 46, 140, 168, 170, 179, 181, 219, 220, 221, 227

outings 3, 12, 27, 82, 119, 150, 160, 206

outreach 148, 149, 150, 151, 152, 153, 154, 155, 159, 160, 161, 162, 163, 164, 165, 166, 210

P

person-centred care 29, 45, 53, 126, 131, 133

photographs 92, 93, 94, 95, 96, 128, 130, 153, 154, 155, 157, 178, 181

profession xv, xviii, xix, 59, 138, 216, 220, 222, 225, 227

Q

quality of life xii, xv, xvi, xviii, 18, 19, 21, 23, 24, 27, 29, 32, 33, 36, 37, 40, 49, 135, 153, 159, 163, 178, 215, 226

R

Registered Homes Act 26, 28, 119

residents and relatives 19, 37, 40, 43, 50, 60, 74, 95, 97, 103, 107, 112, 116, 159, 162, 171, 174, 180, 193, 221, 224

S

supervision 21, 36, 46, 48, 53, 123, 126, 129, 130, 137, 142, 163, 176, 177, 179, 188, 193, 194, 196, 198

V

volunteers 20, 88, 98, 129, 139, 172, 174, 190, 198, 205, 206, 212